fly, my darling

fly, my darling

A LOVE STORY

LISA K. RICHTER

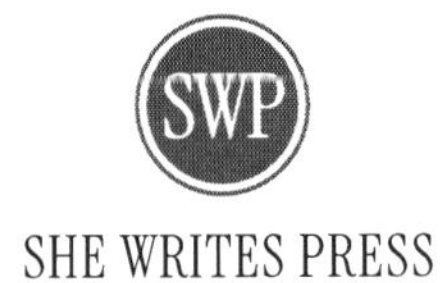

SHE WRITES PRESS

Published in 2026 by
She Writes Press, an imprint of The Stable Book Group

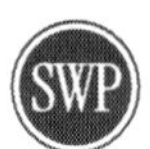

32 Court Street, Suite 2109
Brooklyn, NY 11201
https://shewritespress.com
Library of Congress Control Number: 2025926953
ISBN: 979-8-89636-122-0
eISBN: 979-8-89636-123-7

Interior Designer: Tabitha Lahr

Printed in the United States

Names and identifying characteristics have been changed to protect the privacy of certain individuals.

For Lynda

who promised there is always more.

I know you are listening.

contents

It is okay to be unsure;
we must strive to be brave.

Lucille Clifton,
in conversation,
Olympic Valley, California, 2005

I

Allegro

lively, at a brisk tempo

1.

She stands behind the screen door in the muted light of a cottage shaded beneath banana palms, watching me walk toward her down a short concrete drive. The cottage is tucked within a pod of small beach homes; dense leaves press its green clapboard exterior, wrapping it in more green. A cocoon, I think, eyeing it for the first time.

A vast blue sky, a birdsong afternoon. The air rich with beached sea kelp, salt. When she steps out in jeans and a white tee, a pencil behind her ear, her smile is magnanimous. "Hey there. I'm Lynda." She extends a hand. "You must be Lisa."

Inside, she tidies a composition in progress spread atop a Baldwin grand. In a small side alcove with insulation squares tacked to walls, a double-wide monitor sits above an electronic keyboard, stacks of CDs tower near a standing mic. "Please have a seat." She gestures to a deep leather chair backed against a shelving unit overflowing with music scores and books. A matching sofa in the same worn golden leather and a low pine table fill out the room.

She sits on the piano bench facing me. From the dove-white wall behind her, a framed oil of fiery hues glows. "Where shall we begin?" she says.

2.

I studied classical piano in spurts for some thirty-seven years.

Mrs. Wiley was the first. Arriving at our house Thursdays before dinner, she sat next to me at the antique upright my mother found through an ad in the *Baltimore Sun* and purchased for $60. Mrs. Wiley, with her shiny fingernails and her grandmother voice that never scolded, her repeated exclamations at the aromas wafting from my mother's kitchen, and if it happened to be roast chicken, which it often was on Thursdays, questioning again what made it smell so good, to which I at age seven again and again responded: *rosemary.* There followed more serious classical study through high school. Then after a twenty year pause: Wayne, Madeline, and John, classical concert pianists.

3.

At forty-four, it was time for a new approach, a freer way.

"Call my friend, Lynda," my son's clarinet teacher told me when I mentioned I'd like to try jazz. "I've known her twenty years. She's the one."

4.

She slides off the bench, gestures for me to take her place. “Would you play something?”

I begin the dramatic opening of Beethoven’s *Pathétique* (the French title translating, notably, as both *poignant* and *pathetic*), a composition in classical three-part sonata form.

“Okay,” she says. “That’s good!” Not meaning that it is *good*, but that it is enough. Hands in my lap, I turn to face her. She nods but her body tells all: *Beethoven?*

5.

What is it you want? he pressed me over the years,
the man I'd spent half my life with, *What?*
I didn't have an answer, how could I? It was so big, so much.

When I asked him, *What do you want, what?*
he took a sheet of lined paper and a blue ink pen
and swiftly listed his items, one, two, three, clicked
the pen to retract the ink, dropped it onto the sheet
and looked at it as if to say, Yes, that's it. So easy really.

6.

"Why don't we start here?" She opens a thick, spiral-bound book of jazz standards to "I've Got You Under My Skin."

The musical page is nearly empty. A single note melody line runs beneath clusters of letters and numbers: C7, D9, Eb dim. I have no idea what to do.

"Chord suggestions," she says. She smiles.

7.

“You never are satisfied,” he tells me. “You can have ninety percent of what you want, and still focus on the missing ten percent.” We are walking around the neighborhood—a quiet, gated enclave, manicured, lush with trees. He begins to sprint without me.

Okay. Maybe true. But if that ten percent is the critical amount . . . if what is missing is intangible . . . emotional connection, true intimacy . . . then what?

8.

In the classical realm, perfection is attained by performing a piece as the composer intended. It is all there: each note, phrase, tempo detailed. One knows what one has to do. The difficulty is in the precision, the adherence to the written score.

In jazz, I learn, one needs to challenge the expected, embrace an unscripted page. Its freedom demands an intuitive sense, an unrelenting trust that any sound can be musical.

9.

The mission: Take a simple idea and explore it, using everything you've learned (not nearly enough), and in real time build tone and rhythm, and birth something authentic, moving, beautiful even.

10.

My fingers search for the right notes.
"Let go . . ." she says, standing at my side.

"I'm trying."

She joins me on the bench. Eyes steady on my face, her hands sound a series of melodic, cascading chords.

"Don't *try*. Think only of where you want to land." She plays another run of chords, lingering on the final one. "Like the end of a sigh."

II.

My great-grandfather, on temporary leave from his infantry position in the First World War, was only ten miles away from being reunited with his wife and six children when he learned how the deadly plague had ravaged the family's village. Unable to face what he might find, he returned to the Italian front. His entire family was miraculously still standing, his wife desperate for his strength, for a hand to feed the children, to know whether he was still alive.

My grandfather promised my grandmother a good life in America, just a few years, maybe five, enough to earn something and they would return to Italy. It took twenty years, and then for a visit only. My grandmother hardened to life here in America, hardened to him.

My father, when I was a girl, pulled into the driveway at 5:55 p.m. every workday, Monday through Friday, regardless of hailstorms, hurricanes, or even once a desperate daytime phone call from my housebound mother saying she was done. With it. Forever.

12.

"What was it? What went wrong?" a friend I've known since childhood asks. She believes in my marriage, visited us during our years in Europe, is charmed by him, by what she calls our "worldly life."

I shrug in defeat. It is not one namable thing. Or is it?

"We never really fit," I say. But that isn't it either.

13.

In Italian, there exist two verbs for the English *to know*.

Sapere, to know a fact.
Conoscere, to know a person, a place, a want.

The first involves a binary: yes, no. Do you or don't you?
The second involves full consciousness, familiar connection. Soul.

14.

We sit thigh to thigh on her piano bench, her jeans against my skirt and bare leg. "Like this," she says, dropping her hand in an augmented seventh. It is effortless for her. Harmonies, tonalities, rhythms. "Like this," she says, nodding to me, and I find the shape and rest my hand over hers, my breath trembling, the heady scent of cigarillo floating in her hair.

15.

"Are you pressing keys," she says, "or *allowing the music*?"

"Are you creating sounds . . . or *hearing* them?"

16.

After several months of weekly sessions, I riff for nearly five minutes, improvising a melody, an almost-song.

A mystical pulse fills the room. A musical breakthrough. It seeps into my skin, muscle, heart.

"Yes," she says. Just that: "Yes."

17.

When she was in her mid-twenties, she says, her parents showed up one Saturday evening at the club in New York City, her band's name flashing on the marquee, her father dressed in a plaid bowtie and dark suit, her mother in an A-line dress with pearls, gloves, matching bag and shoes. It was a drunken hole, beer fumes oozing from dirty floorboards. Tats, smoke, a slutty place. They wanted to see what she'd done with her life a year after graduating at the top of her class at Brandeis.

In my mid-twenties, I tell her, newly hired as a programmer in Germany, I discovered that the archdiocese was inhaling a sizable chunk of my salary. Apparently by noting "Catholic" as a religious preference on an employment form, I'd given them the right. When I descended into the building's dank basement and informed the head of personnel that as of that moment I was officially *no longer Catholic*, his face reddened and a gruff voice said, "Sie sind ab sofort kein Gotteskind mehr!" More or less (more) condemning me to German hell. "Okay," I said. "Now where do I sign?"

We laugh,
        and how the room dances.

18.

In a dream, my mother comes back, younger than I remember her, smiling, happy. I know she is here for only a short while, and she knows this, too. She has something important to do. Then she will leave again.

19.

"Leave him," my mother said weeks before she died.

"Mom, it'll be okay," I said, convincing neither of us.

20.

A squally spring wind whistles through the jalousies. After nearly a year, our weekly hour stretches into the afternoon.

A small voice recorder rests on the coffee table. I am documenting her outrageous life.

She begins about an older man and his young mistress, how they follow her from gig to gig—on the Cape, in Boston, western Mass.—study her movements, buy her drinks, hunt her, and eventually proffer a financially lucrative (and creepy) sexual arrangement.

"The woman was hot. A real babe," Lyn winks.

21.

The venue is packed. Guests from the music and arts industry and locals from town gather for the debut of the choral/orchestral work Lyn's been composing for months. She's in high gear, welcoming, introducing. When she sees me standing at the door in a flowing red skirt, a small video camera in hand, she pauses mid-step and whispers my name as if it were holy. She walks toward me, touches my arm, clasps my hand. I raise the camera. "At your service," I say, and we laugh. Someone calls for her. She seems not to hear. When again she whispers my name, the air around us quivers, and I know in that moment on that warm moonless night a year after we met that I will offer myself to her, a carnal desire I've never before imagined or felt for a woman. It is molecular, quantum; there'll be no stopping it.

22.

When she walks off to greet other guests, Andy, a retired LA school teacher and songwriter in his early sixties also studying with Lyn, introduces himself with an endearing smile. "Thank god there's one woman here who isn't a lesbian," he teases. I like him immediately.

23.

I call Lyn the next morning. Can I stop by?

I find the two of them lounging side by side in her rusted patio chairs, smoking, thoughtful.

Andy blows a kiss by my cheek, announces he's off. Lyn touches my arm, her pause says *I'll be right back*, and she walks him to his car.

At the open front window, atop the piano, her cat Zeke turns to me and sings.

> *In composition, it's the outside-octave you aim for. That tone just beyond the one the ear expects to hear. Edgy, it can startle. But add the right note,and it becomes . . . exciting.*

24.

We stand so near her breath finds my lips.
"You are my student. You are married."

"We can't do this," she says.

25.

Occasionally a craving races into my body, not letting on what it is, only that it *is.* After a brief jolt it leaves—allowing moments when I can settle, look at my life and say, *Okay . . .* until the craving comes back.

It always comes back.

26.

I'm wearing a short black skirt, silver heels, and white, scooped tee. A tie emblazoned with piano keys is noosed loosely about my neck. I'm walking the streets, and I can't find it. I stop in a hotel. "Excuse me," to a young, blue-suited woman behind the desk, "can you tell me where the Boom Boom Room is?" She stares at the tie, shakes her head. I retrace my steps to a drab building already passed; darkened glass doors at its corner front and black drapes covering the windows make it a possibility. There's a clatter of laughter, and then I hear her voice. Husky, playful, crooning her "Oxytocin Blues." I pull open the door and stand inside, adjusting to the dim light, the raucous energy. Groups of women press against the room's square bar. Last week she'd said, "Would you like to come? It's Ladies' Night, which means Lesbo Night." She laughed. "You good with that?"

She sits elevated on a mini stage in back, surrounded by her keyboard, amp, speakers, and mic. Our eyes meet and my pulse rages. I haven't yet sorted out how or why or what this might mean. Haven't begun to consider the effects on my marriage, my family tribe. I've told no one, not even myself in an honest way. Mid refrain, "Oxytocin Blues" rolls into a slow, soulful "You Take My Breath Away." The crowd quiets, and bodies turn toward the door, toward me. Andy jumps from a chair at a nearby table with a surprised smile. He calls my name, beckons me over, but Lyn's voice is seduction. The ladies, her friends, sit near her in the back. They wave, their eyes steady as I weave through the bar and join them. A waiter hands me a glass of champagne. "On the house," he says.

Lyn finishes the set and strolls through the room, greeting patrons—remembering names, past conversations.

She takes the seat beside me, leans in. "So glad." The ladies are maybe talking to me, asking. I hear nothing.

In the restroom, musky and dim, she waits near the mirror, her hands cooling under the tap. Her eyes shoot around the small space.

"Oh hell," she says, slamming her back against the door, pulling me to her. My hands find her hair, the cave of her back, her mouth, dark, forbidden.

27.

"Is there more?" My lips at her ear.

"Darling. There is always more."

28.

Jen, a poet friend, is the first one I tell. Jen, who produced erotic recordings of her salacious poetry, who together with her man cast his erect penis in a mold to immortalize it and provide a custom dildo for her ongoing pleasure, who'd gone back and forth between men and women but who now appears hot for a man. Jen, when I tell her, smiles, only mildly shocked. She gives me a long look. "If only I could have been your first," she says.

29.

What is it you want? *What?*

30.

"What do you want to be when you grow up?" Sister enunciated the words as she wrote them in perfect cursive on the green chalkboard. The full-body habit gripping her tired face, she surveyed the grid of small desks: eight rows, five desks each. She began on the left side of the classroom, bouncing her yardstick at one child, then the next. When Kathy said, "I want to be a dancer," most of the class snickered. There were lots of veterinarians. A safe answer. Everyone knew Sister preferred animals to people.

I stared into my lap, watching my fingers stretch out long as twigs. A stench from the room's lunchtime milk crate soured the air. When I looked up, forty sets of eyes looked back. I swallowed, steadied my gaze on Sister's pale impatient face, and listened as a tiny voice said, "Happy."

31.

Lyn sways over the restaurant's Steinway grand, releasing her weight into the chords, a slow, musical sigh. The sound sweeps the room, caresses diners, waiters, the bartender. Voices drop, become intimate. I approach the piano and she returns from a hidden zone, face glowing, conspiratorial. Enormity of her smile.

32.

Several couples drive the ninety minutes down from LA every Saturday to sit at the bar behind her and shout requests. No matter how archaic a tune is, Lyn knows it, and if she doesn't, if they can hum it, she can play it.

One guy—fortyish, built, clean-shaven—routinely buys a bottle of the best champagne, drinks it, and drops a hundred in her tip jar on his way out. As a thank-you, Lyn gallops into something wild and wildly unpredictable, improvised on the spot, once, an ode to Menopause. Men - oh! - Pause.

33.

The Yaris's worn tires screech as they take the corner, the clutch grinding in reverse, backing into the alley behind her cottage where I wait inside with Zeke, he atop the counter, paw pressed to the window, singing nearly five minutes already. *Whao whao whao. . . .* The back door bangs open, keys clang into a dish. Six lunged steps through her kitchen, and she stands energized from the evening's gig, the cat purring smugly around her neck. She nuzzles him, throws me an *I know I know, but if I don't now, he'll never leave us alone* look, then tosses him to the floor and grabs me.

34.

Con abbandono the tempo reads. With abandon.

Meaning, heed no "please slow down."
Meaning, do not rethink, do not look back.
Meaning, on and on you go, a mad acceleration
until that last spectacular note sizzles in the electric air.

35.

"You know," Andy says, "years ago, Lynnie and I sometimes met in town for a drink. We'd talk—about music, twelve-step, the fate of the world, you know—all the while casually scanning the bar. When our eyes settled on the same gorgeous woman, we'd bet who between us would be taking her home."

"And?"

"More I ain't saying."

36.

I invite her to my home for dinner with my kids, my husband. He wants to meet her, to experience directly the woman I speak of so much.

"I took half a Xanax before leaving my place," Lyn emails me later that evening. "When I drove up and saw him waiting in front of your house, I fucking swallowed another."

She was nonstop talking by the time I served the main course. Pumped for a fight, she probably wanted it. It wasn't happening. He was graciously, scarily, maddeningly benign.

37.

Days later, I watch my husband from the front window. He stands in the street with our neighbor, Ted. Their bodies twitch. They are without a doubt bro-bitching about the yapping dogs, the cops speed-ticketing within the community, gates be damned.

"She left me. For a woman," I shamelessly fantasize my children's father saying, though I am inside the house and can hear nothing. "A Jewish lesbian. Smokes cigars. Has the sexiest hair. A tight butt, wit, and a handshake that grabs you right."

Ted hurls spit into the street. A dog begins to bark.

My husband looks down. Slams hands into trouser pockets. "She tried to tell me. And I couldn't be bothered. But . . . [yanks his head swiftly to one side, crack crack] . . . *Christ.*"

38.

Laura, my Jungian analyst, was of my mother's generation, an elegant Peruvian woman with gray-laced auburn hair. "What have you brought today, Lisa?" she'd say, and I'd pass her a copy of what I'd written—vivid recollections of the week's dreams—and read aloud. It was in dreams, Laura said, that one met the truth.

She hadn't a whip of sympathy or hope for my husband, even less for our marriage. "Romance was invented to keep the species procreating."

We sit facing each other in her home's book-filled office. Glass doors look out to a garden of butterfly-laden blossoms and velvet roses. "Look at your kids: beautiful, intelligent, strong. It has less to do with him than with the DNA in the sperm."

Laura leans in, compassionate. "Believe it," she says.

39.

Inside an apartment building in upper Manhattan, I was about to knock on my esteemed piano instructor's door and tell her that I would not be returning, I was unable to focus, too much going on in my life, meaningless excuses but the best I could do because I was forty and restless and I didn't know why I would not be coming back. We would be moving again in a couple months. It was what my husband wanted. It was not what I wanted, not what the children wanted.

The hall elevator opened and a woman and young girl emerged. The girl was four, maybe five, dressed in a pastel blue coat, white socks, and shined black Mary Janes. A mini navy purse dangled in her hand. In an Easter photo taken when I was four, I wear a wool coat of the same dust blue, the same black patent shoes, those limp curls at my face. I, too, once had a small leather purse. The girl stopped, even as the woman continued toward the building's exit.

"Who are you?" she said. We faced each other in the narrow hall, openly staring. Who are you? deep in her eyes a moment more before she sprang out the building into the white sky.

40.

"She Will Fly" is the first song Lyn writes and records for me.

The song ends. Then after a couple beats of silence there begin breathless exclamations; Lyn's voice changes to project several "bystanders" staring up into the sky.

> *Wow! Look at her go!*
> *Yeah, man. She's flyin!*

41.

"I'd give anything to do what you do," he tells Lyn when she stops performing for a break, this midlife guy, a never-tipper regular at her gig in Newport Beach, hanging at the edge of the bar, a breath from her keyboard. "Quit my job, stop *working*, just play music evenings in a place like this."

I am watching, hearing, from a nearby table. I can tell she's had enough. "You know," she says, "there's a lot of study and practice and slog that goes into this, into making it look effortless."

He smiles. He shouldn't have.

"Tell you what," Lyn says. "Let's switch. You take my gigs and my twenty-year-old Toyota, and I'll take whatever the hell it is you do and the keys to the Benz you drove in here."

He scratches a perfectly trimmed sideburn. Turns toward the bartender, wiggles his empty glass.

42.

A howl vibrates along the wall. I panic, wondering if it might be my husband closed upstairs in the bedroom we have shared, grieving the loss, a future taken for granted as the foundation of his tomorrow. A future, I told him days before, I could no longer be a part of.

I go to the window, lift the sash. A moment of thick silence, then I hear it. A neighbor's hound. Heart-stopping loneliness flung into the night.

43.

"He loves you, you know," a friend says, sipping her iced vodka. "It's splashed all over that pouty, funereal visage of his. That and, really, he can't figure out why you're leaving his dick [pause] for a woman." She sucks in an ice cube, spits it back into her glass. "Why the hell are you?"

"I'm not leaving him for a woman," I say. "I'm leaving him for Lynda."

44.

Two middle-aged saleswomen greet me from behind the glass counters in a small jewelry store near the old Capistrano mission, a sparkling sea of turquoise and silver before them. I stretch out my left hand, point to the ring, and explain.

The women lean in to hear. Tiny wrinkles flash at their eyes. "I'm with you," one says, slipping the clipper beneath the simple band I've not removed in twenty-three years, her hands steady as the gold springs apart. A shocked stillness, as if three hearts in that moment forget to thump.

The next day my fifteen-year-old son taps the bare finger, a pale circle remaining on my skin. His wise face, crushed.

45.

"Coraggio, Lisa, coraggio." Magda leaned close, gripping my hand. The room with its ceiling-high windows, the bed blanketed in white. A wooden cross nailed above the door.

La Quiete (The Calm), the private clinic—a magnificent villa above Varese—where my son would be born.

"Oggi nasce un miracolo," Magda, blessed midwife, promised as the contractions gained in intensity, tumbling one upon the other. Hour after hour she calmly encouraged, then raised her voice with mine when I began to shout.

46.

Coraggio, I write, large letters, on a found scrap of worn cardboard,
a remnant from that final cross-country move four years ago,
the one I told his dear parents who sat then in the kitchen with me
sipping coffee as I peeled potatoes, that after nineteen years together
and already eight moves, three of them international, that this one might
possibly be the end to everything.

47.

We float in a shined black vessel, my husband and I hovering at opposite ends, our daughter and son filling the hollow between.

"Here is Dante's house," Marco, grinning in striped white and black, says with a pull of the gondola's oar. But it is not his house, I know; Dante stayed only briefly in Venice while passing through. Marco tells stories as if they are truths. Directing our journey, he is charming, stupid.

Can he not tell there is no love?

Approaching the bridge, he says, "When we pass under, you must kiss each other, all couples must. It is tradition in my city."

My man swaggers to me (*Un bacio per l'amore eterno!*) though I've said it is over, though he knows I can't.

He throws his muscle around me, his mouth to mine. On my thigh a pat-pat-pat: There, see, *you can.*

We glide beneath the bridge, Il Ponte dei Sospiri, the famed crossing named for the expired breaths of prisoners as they walked from light to dungeon and watched hope's last glow snuff out.

48.

In front of me: *The Titanic Days*, by René Magritte. A rape, a nude woman fighting off a man. Except, Magritte has drawn them as one person. Is this because the man has invaded her completely—entered her, become part of her? His savage hands have her waist, her thigh. Or is this an interior battle: man, woman. A mortal raping of the innocent self, the beautiful one. Horrified, I wander by it twice, then take off, exposed.

49.

When I open the screen door, Lyn is on the phone with a stranger she called from a DNC list hoping to turn votes for Obama, her blond curls combed to a froth, the sleeves of her red flannel shirt folded back. She ends the call.

"Not sure I convinced her," she says. "The woman is set on McCain. But! I've just learned—in detail—how to prepare her abuela's famous chicken liver mash." No one hangs up on Lynda. It's the way she says hello.

She slides her pencil behind her ear. Gives me a good stare. "Okay. Shoes off, bag down." A mug of mint tea finds its way into my hands and she disappears. I sip the tea, ruminating on my life, all that isn't working, so much beyond my control to fix. The minutes slip away.

She leads me to the bathroom, a room not much larger than a closet and with two doors so that it serves as a walk-through at the back of the cottage. The yellow floor tiles gleam. A fresh towel hangs over the edge of the old cast-iron tub filling with water. She tosses in a handful of Epsom salts and rose petals which she must have plucked from the shrubs out back (an extravagance, I imagine, she rarely allows herself). A small painted cabinet with a mirror hangs above a miniature white pedestal sink framed in blush and black tiles. Built into the wall is a heater, an authentic, circa 1930s unit, pulsing warm air into the room. Steam condenses on the mirror. White candles balancing on the sink's lip illuminate the room. By the time I sink into the warm water, life begins to settle again. Lyn is back at the piano, improvising a ballad, another in the series of her choral project.

She returns. I rise from the bath, and she wraps me in a towel. When she finally speaks, her voice is grave but gentle.

"Lisa," she says, "just be yourself. It'll make life a whole lot easier."

50.

Tikkun olam:
The Jewish mitzvah of healing the world.

"When Lynda spoke," a childhood friend of hers from their Temple youth group tells me, "we listened."

51.

"Who's number one?" Lyn says.

"I am."

"Who?"

"Me."

"Louder!"

"I AM."

"Louder!"

"I AM!"

"Say it . . ."

"I AM NUMBER ONE."

"Yes you are, darling," she says. "Don't ever forget it."

52.

Deb, Lyn's first genuine love and bandmate for years, has invited me to her apartment. She's curious about me and I, her.

"Lynda was wearing red platform shoes when we met," she tells me, laughing, her blond shag and deep bangs reminiscent of the '70s. I laugh too, knowing it must be true, picturing it however unlikely, wanting to have been there, then.

They left Boston, she says, and drove across the country in a used Volkswagen Rabbit. "All we did when we got to LA was take our clothes off. We went to the nude beaches. Got jobs nude modeling."

Opening a folder of memorabilia, she reveals more of their story, of the gigs in Atlantic City and Vegas. The year is 1978. I smell the sweet-sour smoke of pot and tobacco. Beer, perfume. Hear heels and boots clomping across a wooden dance floor. Deb on stage, swinging her guitar, the bass screaming thump, thump, thumpthump. Big hair, spandex, gold bangles. Lyn pounding her double keyboards, "I Feel the Earth Move," belting the lyrics.

53.

"So, Lisa-baby," Lyn's lawyer friend, Sid, a large woman with enormous heart, says when we find ourselves alone after word gets out that Lyn and I are a couple, "tell me, yeah, tell me about it. The first time." When she focuses intently, the New Yawker comes out thick and loud. "I mean, ya made changes in ya life recently, but this, I mean this is fuckin' over the top." She wraps me in her arms, pulls me into her generous flesh.

54.

"You have some weird friends, Mom," my daughter says.
"Probably because I'm weird myself."
"True," she says. "But in a good way."
"You know, you've some weird friends, too," I say.
"I guess. But nothing like yours."

55.

"Listen, Mom. California is probably a good place for you," she says. "You've got people here that support you. I mean, really, where else could you leave a man for a woman and have everyone be generally okay with it? California is good. Think if you lived on the East Coast. Or in Europe. *God*."

56.

Born in a small village hospital in southwest Germany, my daughter entered life perfect: dark hair, button lips, flawless skin, eyes calm and alert.

I'd shared a maternity room with a local woman whose extended family and friends were a constant presence during visiting hours. They chatted and laughed, loud bodies curled around her bed, and regarded me curiously: What was a young American woman doing here—alone?

And who, some surely then wondered, was the business-suited man who stopped by briefly in the evenings after work to nuzzle the newborn before disappearing again? Father of the child? Husband? Why didn't he comfort the woman, bring her books, music, some decent food? Why didn't he stay longer?

57.

Andy calls. *Meet me at 10 at the coffee pub!* When I arrive, he hugs me, shakes his head. "You. And Lynnie." He adds with a smile, "What are you now, my favorite lesbian?" There is no sexual bridge for him, no energy to consider.

58.

“How do you do that?” he asks. “How do you kiss another woman?”

“How do you not?”

59.

She lounges on her side, skin to sheet, watching me undress, waiting for me, not ravenous, not yet . . . allowing the tender moment. One arm lies beneath a cascade of loose curls, the other in front of her, palm up, her lips softly closed. It is her body which speaks. *We've all afternoon*, it says. *This will happen at your speed.*

The blue armoire along one wall. The filtered jalousie light. Sounds from the street, from the neighbor sweeping her patio just feet from the bedroom, listening in.

When our bodies first touch, she heaves a sigh, intense, lusty, exhilarated, and I think: *This is enough.* Just this, this body to body, skin to skin. If there is nothing more in life, ever, *this* will be enough.

60.

Beneath us, enveloping us: an intoxicating fluff of flannel and down.

Making music is like making love, she explains. You can tell when musicians blend: A groove is established and all the invisible cues go floating. They follow the same unheard dynamics, instinctively knowing when one wants to take the lead with a solo, when the tempo should pick up, when it will wind down, which instrument will have the last note, and what that note will be.

61.

There's only two ways to sum up music. Either it's good or it's bad. If it's good you don't mess about it, you just enjoy it.

Louis Armstrong

62.

"The lesbo scene can be incestuous." Lyn adds another scoop of cucumber salad to the broiled halibut on her plate. I pour myself a second glass of merlot and wait for her to continue. "Especially where the pickings are few, when the town is small. Eventually everyone does it with everyone else, or almost." She rattles off the names of women who are now also my friends. X was together with Y, then Y with Z, then X with Z, and then there was K who'd enjoyed a couple men lately, too. Before Lyn was with me, she was with an artist, creator of the oils dressing her walls. And before that a female golf star. And before that . . . well, there were many. Lyn brings me to the brink of that world, close enough to peer in. Opens the gate wide for me to enter, but I straddle the doorway, a foot on either side.

63.

A former neighbor approaches me in the checkout at Whole Foods. She taps me on the shoulder and looks me up and down three times with a frozen smile.

64.

They begin falling away. The images of me, of who they thought I was, the perfect one, the one with the career, the family, the husband, the one who had it all together. They are falling away, like an undressing of Gustav Klimt's sad Adele, lost in all those golden robes.

65.

Adele Bloch-Bauer's wealthy husband commissioned Klimt to paint her in elaborate brocade gowns so he could splash his wealth across foyer walls, wanting to impress visitors with how he idolized her. Adele and Klimt engaged in a secret affair, and Klimt painted her exquisite, seductive face on many nudes as well, though her husband never saw these. Or if he did, remarked at how his goddess's face so resonated with the artist that he felt compelled to employ it again. Secretly this delighted Adele's husband—that he possessed something of such inestimable value.

66.

"I don't think you'll be needing that IUD anymore," Lyn says several months into our relationship, a year and a half after we met. Meaning, get rid of it, girl. We sprawl in shorts on the leather sofa, end to end, facing each other. Zeke naps against our legs, a languid, rolling purr. I tell her then. About that sickening evening. I'd been a virgin. So long ago.

67.

I'm having a party, he said, New Year's Eve.

I was twenty
dressed for a gala
expecting others to arrive
expecting a celebration.
A beaten house lit by a lone weak bulb
the door buzzed a warning
        my innocence didn't hear.
He popped open a beer
swigged it dry then passed it to me
a proud high school grad
a stocker in a sporting goods store.
It was his profile I'd once admired,
a Romanesque nose, aristocratic.
He hummed "Heaven Must Have Sent You"
swaying left and right
staring into the emptiness behind me.

~

What was wrong with that girl
so desperate for love
so wanting to be good

that she didn't hate him?
not then
not when the clinic told her the impossible news
not when she told him and a handful of lies
    dripped like "pings" in a cold metal bucket
not when she wept over the rush of blood
not until the bastard called, two years later.
Hey, what's up? he said.

It took years to try to forget.
There was no forgetting.

"Fucking shithead," Lyn says as she holds me. Her embrace says: Use it. Let it keep you strong.

68.

At the family farmhouse north of Venice, my grandmother's brother climbed a hand-nailed ladder to the rafters and plucked a wispy-feathered young pigeon from a nest, holding her gently within his callused hands.

Zio Paolo wanted to show me, because I asked, how to prepare his sauteed squab. Olio, he told me, rosmarino, aglio.

My daughter, not yet two, ran in the front garden, peering into rabbit cages, chatting with innocent beauties destined to become coniglio arrosto before the year was out. Her brother, soon to be born, heavy within me.

Paolo slid thumb and forefinger around the bird's neck, explaining a few seconds is all you need. His fingers tightened momentarily; I held my breath and shook my head.

Innocent. Taken.

He let go and the babe opened her beak—a gasp—and quivered. Slice here, Paolo told me, still squeezing the handful of pale gray fluff. He showed where to make the incision to remove the innards. The gizzard. The liver. The tiny tiny heart.

69.

Lyn finds a poem fragment. "May I read it?"

A rolling landscape. Bright flowers
in stone vases. Metal plates flush in the ground.
My mother lay suspended in a carved box,
wood shined and smoothed and perfect.
How she had wanted her life to be.
How she had hoped my life would be.
Morning's calm blew into a bitter wind.
My black lace flapped. The tented canopy rose, then
snapped. Trees whirled and wailed in a beseech
for love as young spring leaves clung on.
I shivered. Bones blood flesh cold.
The undertaker's son saw, came,
slipped from suit jacket thick with aftershave
tobacco sweat
draped me in its warmth,
remained by my side.

She lifts her eyes from the page to my face. Removes her glasses. Being heard. It can be everything.

70.

. . . When a girl screams in nighttime terrors, her mother's solution is not to discuss the fear, but rather blanket the bedroom's walls in sunshine yellow and paint overtop a cheerful girl in a white-pearled blouse and hooped skirt surrounded by ducklings and daisies and a gentleman suitor bowing and lifting his hat. She gushes over the mural, wanting for her daughter so much, though she knows—as do you—there is no comfort in fairy tales.

71.

. . . And if she excels in math, then that's what she will do,
not writing, but mathematics,
because how many girls are actually good in math?
You will have a stable job with good pay.
You have a future ahead of you,
because you are pretty,
because you can work with numbers,
because you can think like a man.

72.

In *How Not to Be Wrong*, mathematician and writer Jordan Ellenberg relates the following dilemma. During WWII, when American war planes returned from Europe, they were ridden with bullet holes, many more in the fuselage, few in the engine. For efficiency, the military wanted to reinforce the areas where the planes were hit the hardest, asking how much more armor was needed to pad the fuselage.

Abraham Wald, a mathematician, knew that statistically the bullet holes should have been more uniformly spread over the plane. *You need to focus on the missing bullet holes*, Wald said. Because they were on the missing planes. A plane shot in the engine wasn't coming back. It was simple: The armor needed to go where the bullet holes *weren't*.

73.

Visiting my parents, on break from college, sometime around midnight: a girl's smothered scream, a car door slamming. Then nothing.

I rapped on my parents' bedroom door, cracked it open. "Dad." I explained. "She needs help."

He said, "Go back to sleep."

In my childhood room, I sat at an open window terrified that I would hear something, terrified that I wouldn't, wondering if I'd really heard what I was certain I had, how she was surviving it.

74.

Five years after my mother died, I stand at her grave with my father. The final months his doctor gave him have run out. It will be his last visit before he is in the ground with her, and he knows it.

I kneel next to him stifling a desperate sob as he yanks at weeds. Cleaning, tidying. It is his prayer.

When we leave, we cross Baltimore to the cemetery where his mother, father, and sister are—his family—so that I will know, will remember, will from time to time visit their graves too, will pass it on.

75.

Right off, I hear the music, see Lyn dancing beyond the front window. Headphones on, twirling, swaying, such inner joy. I slow my approach. She sees me, flies to the computer, shuts it down. Eyes flash. "You're early!"

Weeks later I receive the recording, "You Knew All Along," her own, a bossa nova rhythm spilling the incredulity of our love.

Just like night and day
we lead different lives
Somehow we still see eye to eye

A poem or a song
reminds us we belong
Together until the end of time.

76.

"Mathematics," Jordan Ellenberg wrote, "is the study of things that come out a certain way because there is no other way they could possibly be."

77.

I smell the Pacific's mist flowing in, landing on the pine table, a salty film that will attract a layer of dust by morning. Hear the cottage creek, a clink of the Scotch bottle, a rattle of ice. The leather sofa releases a moan, then another. She is outstretched, I know, in her striped boxers. Her breath pulses into the phone, mine pulses back, a continent away. I am in the basement of my sister's home. Breath to breath, long into the night, she stays with me, holding me steady. My father is gone, buried on my forty-sixth birthday.

78.

. . . When you are young, the answer to death is simple: Dig out a rectangle; shovel in the carcass; cover with pebbles and dirt; finish with a feisty stomp. The cemetery should be an impressive four foot square. A brick surround, twig crosses thatched together with twine. Each small creature, domestic or wild, laid to rest with a headstone. Blueberry, Snippy, Igor . . . crayoned in white. When Mr. Gray, the new neighbor who stole the adjoining woods lot, discovers the headstones while walking behind his home and approaches your mother with his Washingtonian stockbroker twit, "My dear, I believe there may be a burial ground on my property? Some cross markings and bricks with names?" your mother, sensing your hidden perch above in the sycamore tree, will answer, "Not to worry, Mr. Gray. I'm sure each deceased was given a thoughtful burial. Some rats, if I recall, a pair of parakeets. A few toads." Then as Gray fidgets and pales, your mother will drop her voice, the drama!, "And poor, bushy Harold, the hellion, pancaked by the mail truck. . . ."

79.

"I want to grow old with you," I say.

"Hell, darling, we're already old."

"Oh fuck it. Then I want to grow older with you."

80.

I am in her kitchen with its original built-in wooden cabinetry, yellow antique range, large ceramic sink surrounded with black tile. Retro, classic, it could be truly spectacular if Lyn had an interest in renovating. But she doesn't have an interest, or the finances, or time for the past.

We are spending the day together, trying out what it might be like to share a home. She is in the adjoining room, at her piano, composing a mini opera to *Uncle Tom's Cabin*. Complex, atonal sounds. Suddenly she stands in the kitchen doorway. "I like squash, too," she says as I add another smashed tear of garlic to a pan of sizzling zucchini and sweet onion. A patient smile. "But darling, it's three in the afternoon. Don't you have some writing to do?"

81.

Though George's and Eliza Harris's words exist in separate chapters in *Uncle Tom's Cabin*, Lyn brings them together in a love duet she titles "Free." The two affirm their perilous connection in a way that Harriet Beecher Stowe likely never imagined. It is a requiem to love, to its fragility, challenge, its everlasting spirit after earthly defeat.

82.

Art must always come first, she reminds me later. The connection to the beautiful which transcends. It is how we survived.

83.

Lyn knows her emotional limit, and a once-a-week drive to her dad at a Jewish care home in Los Angeles is it. Before visiting with him, she opens the grand piano parked in the hub of the end-of-life ward where hallways intersect, and begins. Cole Porter, Ella Fitzgerald, Billie Holliday, Nina Simone. Residents peek from their rooms and find their way toward her, a steady stream of leisure wear and bathrobes and slippers. They hum or sing along, the sudden light in their faces crushingly beautiful, reinforcing Lyn's certainty that music breathes in the soul and is never forgotten, even when all else is.

On one occasion, her father sits listening in a wheelchair, tapping his fingers, his deep voice anticipating every word of every verse, he one of the few in a collared shirt, sometimes even topped with one of his signature bow ties. "She's quite good," I overhear him tell the nurse standing at his side. "Who is she?"

84.

Weeks later her father grabs her, calls her by her mother's name, tries to kiss her. Where has she been! The disease is progressing. No one has told him that his wife died more than a year ago, certain the grief will rupture his already fragile mind.

"Just shoot me," Lyn says, her voice gnarled as we pull out of the assisted living lot, the Toyota's gear grinding as it maneuvers a crazed swerve into dense traffic. "You hear? When the time comes. Take me out." Her face is pale, her body steeled. She drops into third and floors it through a yellow.

"She's the smartest person I know," her friend David told me on a recent visit from his home in Hartford, Connecticut. He's as liberal and irreverent as Lyn, and he's known her nearly fifty years.

Certainly, losing her mind, the ability to reason and create, would violate Lyn to the core. But take her from her life, from mine? I crack the window, stare at a florescent sky. *Don't ask this of me.*

Lyn loosens her knuckled grip of the wheel. She's already moved on. Occasionally, she times herself: five minutes to bitch and cry and then enough. Back to the day, the work at hand. She modifies this philosophy somewhat for me when I blubber, allowing me initially the time I think I need. Then just as I am about to be tarred by all that is unconscionably wrong, she'll slap me with a firm but loving, "Okay, time to let go, more will be revealed," and get up and fold laundry or make us tea. She has the grit to stop me cold.

The Toyota gradually finds a steady speed. We cruise toward home beneath the afternoon summer sun, the traffic all but gone. Along Coast Highway pedestrians cluster on corners heaving beach chairs, umbrellas, coolers. A young boy, trim bronze body, wobbles a surfboard on his head.

85.

When Lyn was young, her father, she told, would on occasion bring her and her sister into the master bedroom walk-in closet and close the door, trapping them in darkness. With a small flashlight, he removed a shoebox from the upper shelf and, slowly prying the lid, removed photos of relatives who'd succumbed during the Holocaust. Black-and-white images gray in the dim glow. He told the same simple story each time. Lyn's sister cowered behind her, digging fingers into Lyn's back.

Everyone in Lyn's family was dark haired: her sister, brother, parents, cousins. Lyn is blond, blue-eyed. Which made those terrorizing closet episodes all the more frightful. Would she have been left behind, with everyone she loved sent to the camps? It wasn't until her niece had a daughter, another blond blue-eyed girl, that she stopped wondering about the authenticity of her genes.

86.

I meet her extended family for the first time at her father's burial. "This here is my darling," Lyn says with an arm around me, then walks off. All eyes, they size me up. Cousins, niece, nephew, aunts, uncles: community activists, doctors, lawyers, professors, Hebrew scholars, art historians. A family of purpose.

Their smiles are genuine; serious but not unkind. "Lisa, what do you do?"

I stumble. "I'm applying to a master's program. . . ."

> Do? I craze-spin, that's what, trying to keep my family together while loving your Lynda, and failing. These days I know nothing of nothing, I am torn, and your simple question in this moment is shredding me.

Their earnest attention waits, hopes for more. Lyn returns to my side. "Lisa is a poet, a writer," she says. And they nod, maybe satisfied, maybe just polite, relieved to move on.

87.

"I don't want to know what you *do*," my female protagonist says to a potential love interest she approaches in a bar. "*Tell me what you ache for.*"

88.

Geometry had always been my favorite discipline. A visual math composed of straight and curvaceous lines, its axioms allow for a stepwise progression to a decisive conclusion, the solving of a dilemma. Solid, satisfying, the answer always there, waiting to be found.

89.

The gift is waiting for me bedside when I awake in her cottage. Simply wrapped in manuscript paper, it's a collection of Brahms piano pieces. A gorgeous Henle edition. Iconic pale blue binding, heavy ivory-toned pages.

March 28. 08
For Lisa –
On your 47th birthday –
With Love
Lyn

A Post-it note on page 86 flags where the composition begins, the *Intermezzo in A*, the classical piece I heard the first time just weeks ago, the one I told her I wanted to learn, had to learn, the music almost too beautiful.

I hear her in her kitchen, dicing apples for our breakfast. The aroma of steeping coffee. My daughter is moving to Berkeley in the fall. My son is remaining with his father. I am leaving them. My husband, willingly. My daughter and son, my heart tells me unforgivably.

I slide my fingers over the music, feeling the melody, asking for forgiveness.

Intermezzo. A brief interlude, a diversion.
Andante teneramente. To be performed at a moderate tempo, with tenderness.

90.

After silence, that which comes nearest to expressing the inexpressible is music.

Aldous Huxley

91.

A year later, I rent a small home of my own, a five minute walk from Lyn's. Near the beach, in town. A storybook cottage with wood and terracotta flooring, a rustic fireplace, large windows that leak with every rain. I buy a bed, bring a table—once prominent in my grandfather's workshop—now my writing desk, a chair, and boxes of books.

Slowly, slowly, I move from the house where I lived for years, the nest where my children grew, where my parents spent time, where we all once laughed. My daughter away at college, my son is home, silently watching me dismantle his stability. *How does he endure that? How? How do I?*

I remember standing in the open living room, he leaning over the upstairs railing looking. Just the two of us in the house, his father traveling. I don't remember saying anything.

I take a few extra things: my grandmother's fine dishware, a cherished pan I'd brought back from Italy, my Bialetti espresso pot. When I eventually send my piano to my rented cottage, I'm not sure any of us will survive it.

92.

Why was I not more joyful? Lyn insists. This was to be *our* time.

She challenges me, forces me to take a stand, strikes flint against stone. "You must for once think of yourself, Lisa. Think of us."

"I don't think she'll ever accept it," a close friend and practicing therapist says to me, "the active, inseparable bond you have with your children, that you belong to a loving tribe separate from her, in addition to her. She's never been a mother, and from the moment she could escape her home, her childhood, she did, and never looked back."

Her expression acknowledges the depth of the dilemma. "She wants *you*. All of you."

93.

In the ER. A tiny non-room, a white curtain on a metal bar enclosing the cot on which Lyn semi-reclines and the plastic chair on which I sit, cell in hand, checking texts, the day filled with activity. Am I worried? she wants to know.

"About what?"

There is the impending divorce, decisions to be made, so much to sort through, my sister arriving at the airport to help.

There is, too, the urgent hunt for a home for Lyn and me to share, the realtors texting moments ago: They've found something promising, if we want it we'll need to move fast, meet them in an hour?

And then the completion of my degree, the senior reading I am to give, the seminar I am soon to teach. . . .

"Worried," Lyn says. "About this cramp."

It's the reason we are sitting here, waiting for an ultrasound of her leg. I shake my head looking at her, glowing and muscular, at the gym yesterday deadlifting 220 pounds. She watches her cholesterol, eats lots of greens, lean protein, swallows a handful of vitamins daily. Worried?

II

Adagio

slowly, with great expression

94.

Lyn insists there's a mix-up. I feel nothing, think nothing. Only: This is happening to someone else. She calls our friend Michele. The phone pressed to her ear, still I hear Michele shriek, begin a full-out wail.

Lyn keeps saying, "They've made a mistake, they've made a mistake."

95.

The stool wobbles as he shifts his weight. Behind him, opaque curtain. A space too small for such cruelty.

He stays less than a minute, standing up when he has just sat down. Slick, dark hair. A body in a white coat. A voice with no face.

96.

I've some unfortunate news. Is that it? Is that what he says? Or does he say, "We have the results. Cancer. Seriously metastasized. We'll arrange a room for you upstairs."

97.

What is it you want? *What?*

98.

There's a spare bed in the room, but I lie next to her the first night, sharing her pillow, her cotton blanket, pulling myself on the skinny mattress not to wake her. In the morning, after little sleep, I whisper from a tear-swollen face, "What will I possibly do, how will I make it without you?"

When I was young and monsters hugged my bed, I'd race to my parents' room and slip in when their door was unlocked, which was not always, and seek my mother's warmth, lying at the edge of the mattress against her stomach, barely a breath, praying to be allowed to stay.

Lyn is warm—a slight fever—and I hold her, hold the heat of her body against the cool of my own. "Don't lay that on me, darling. I don't need the guilt trip," she says. Someone in the hall moves a cart, its rattle jars the morning calm. A screech of rubber-soled shoes, a sigh of tedium from a nightshift nurse longing for the eight hours to end. "We'll get through this," she says, blue eyes alertly pensive. There is something at work within her; prayer, yes, but something more. I begin to slide from the bed. She guides her hand under my shirt, along my spine, and pulls me in.

99.

"We had so many plans," I tell Andy in the hospital room when he arrives, shaking his head, Lyn away for another scan, the news one day old. I tell him again in the hallway. In the elevator. While in line for coffee downstairs. Each time he wraps me in a hug, holds on. I tell him my mother died from the same lung cancer eight years ago. Five young grandchildren she was just getting to know. She was only seventy-two. Images of the future fall away, petals dropping in clumps from a ripe, perfect blossom. Lyn is fifty-eight.

100.

Lyn's brother Sam, 6'3", hair buzzed short-short, arrives jovial, darkly handsome in his casual polo shirt, gripping a Starbucks latte. Despite the fact that he is fifteen years younger—or maybe because of it—the two have a special affection for each other. He's flown in from New York, staying nearby with a friend while I stay in-room with Lyn—she, too, revved up this morning, having dreamed through the night's interruptions of blood pressure checks and IV refills, aided by a generous dose of Ativan. Sam's booming voice fills the room as they kid around, certain the situation isn't serious. Friends parade in, arms laden with organic granola, apples, books. Glances swing from Lyn to Sam to me, lingering on me.

It's Sunday, and I've been wearing the same clothes for days. My hair unwashed. When was the last time I brushed my teeth?

101.

Another friend strolls in, joins the room's lively crowd. She turns and scrutinizes the wooden crucifix just above the door, Jesus dangling, red splats on his face, chest, and palms. "Now that's uplifting," she says and takes a paper plate from Lyn's untouched lunch, draws a Star of David, asks a nurse aide to give her a boost, and covers the crucifix with the star. A round of applause.

Something in my Catholic gut objects, but only briefly.
It's a frightening image: an innocent being, ravaged, lost to circumstances beyond his control.

102.

Lyn and a Russian nurse have been discussing existential philosophy for nearly an hour. It's not yet 9 a.m. Gurdjieff, Ouspensky, *The Fourth Way.* Lots of ponderous spirituality. I studied Ouspensky some years ago, but I don't join in.

All I can do is this: breathe in, breathe out.

A murder of crows swoop-lands on a near branch.
A spread of black feathers, and they are gone.

103.

"There is not a single useful negative emotion," P. D. Ouspensky in his lecture collections is quoted as saying. "Sacrifice your suffering."

104.

"Try to understand the meaning of *silence* in the work, the meaning of *sincerity*, and the meaning of *truth*," Ouspensky offers. "We . . . must see where we can change something, because . . . there is always a point where it is possible to begin."

105.

Lyn sits on her front patio, reading the *New York Times*, coughing, coughing. The hospital released her after six days, sent her home with an oxygen tank and rounds of happy hugs. Her friend David, who flew from Hartford when he heard the news and is staying in my cottage, tells me he's been perusing my *New Yorker* magazines piling up untouched on a side table. "There is an interesting article," he says scratching his beard, "about a woman with lung cancer and the ongoing hope the doctors and everyone sent her way, because they had to, because it was the way they—the doctors and family—managed the unmanageable, avoided the reality. And how . . . Well, you read it," he says. "Maybe not now. Maybe it's too much now. But Lisa, you need to read it."

106.

"Hey, hon," Lyn says when I dance into the cottage waving a fistful of bright helium balloons and a bottle of champagne. Hours earlier she celebrated the prayed-for news: The hospital sent word that the liver biopsy confirmed she was a match for a new targeted gene therapy, a miracle cure that would wipe out the cancer. *Gone.* The beast annihilated.

Her face is solemn. "They got it wrong."

An oncologist reviewing the data realized the mistake and the hospital called again. You see because the disease began in the lung not in the liver somehow the cancer was a different cancer and although one set of cells matched it was not the right set of cells and they could schedule a biopsy of lung tissue and yes they would do that anyway it should have been done at first maybe it had already? It wasn't clear who wrongly authorized the liver biopsy or how or why but no there was no available targeted therapy or well there might be but realistically the chances were basically none and ~

107.

Lyn wrote a two-page letter and mailed over forty pages of medical records to the Gonzalez clinic in New York, an innovative cancer center hailed as the answer. A week later, we hear back. The response is received by email.

Thank you for your interest. We don't believe we can help you.

108.

She asks me to get her a bat. Not one of those kiddy smurf ones. The real thing: solid wood with a good grip. "It's time to vent, bust some shit up," she says.

109.

Wound to heal. This kind woman, a credentialed holistic physician in Los Angeles, offers the words with clear irrefutability.

Wound to heal, you've got to do it. Sounds like a line from a Stones' tune. Scare the cancer, she said, shake it up, shake it out. Then flood the body with good stuff. She shares stories of miraculous healings. "It is The Way," she says, and Lyn and I are willing believers.

There will be regular chemotherapy along with a brown powder of crushed turkey rhubarb, burdock root, slippery elm bark, and other pulverized organic matter steeped overnight in distilled water, dried medicinal mushrooms, lemon grass, asparagus.

110.

Research finds that burdock root (*gobo* in Japanese) in particular, offers promising inhibitory effects on cancer cell growth. It contains arctigenin, a lignan which stops the production of certain proteins, restricting cancer's ability to reproduce. The root is known to purify blood, strengthen the lymphatic system, act as a natural diuretic, heal the skin, lower blood sugar, treat enlarged spleens, and fight tonsillitis. It is, potentially, also an aphrodisiac.

III.

Eve sits on the rug, leaning against the sofa, munching from a bowl of leftovers she found in the fridge. She and Lyn have known each other for years. Sixty and attractive (sexy, Lyn once offered), she is sharing about the men in her past, the current emptiness she feels. She is still looking, hoping.

I'm in the kitchen opening a bottle of wine when I hear Lyn, silent for some time, ask her: What is it you really want?

I hand Eve a glass of Chianti and join Lyn on the sofa. Eve sips, studying us, thoughtful. "I want what you have," she says.

"How did I get so lucky," Lyn says as I wind my fingers through hers. Eve leans in closer and Lyn begins to quietly sing a swooning "Fly Me to the Moon," and the heaviness lifts. There is love, so much love, and I am carried. I am floating, away.

112.

Our last married moments together, my husband and I sit in a small office conversing in gentle tones. He in a denim shirt and khakis, I in a simple dress of pale blue. I sign the settlement first, then he—a flourish, last name only, after so many years in America, still a German—the attorney watching us, her face sullen, her eyes saying don't, don't throw it away, you are making a mistake, which is perhaps true, but it is too late, it has maybe always been too late, for us, for all we didn't know those years ago, for the unraveling that happened in between. At fifty-seven he is as lean as he was at thirty-one, though he had hair then, curls flipping at his neck, wide-bottomed linen trousers dancing when he walked, pale socks, dark European loafers, a pronounced accent, the early beginnings of what became an unshakable ambition.

Things come apart, my look to her, equally sullen, says.

113.

Todd McLellan's tall book filled with mind-boggling photographs sits on a shelf in my room. *Things Come Apart: A Teardown Manual for Modern Living.* "The waste and expense of having to replace everything in your life after just a few years of use is exasperating," he writes. "The teardown movement challenges our disposable culture by exposing just what we are throwing away. . . . [Objects] were repaired when broken, not discarded." He has photographed his disassembled objects first laid out in the order in which their singular pieces were revealed, a precise and formal image. And then, after setting them free, he captures them in pure free fall.

What McLellan fails to mention is that a teardown can expose irreparable damage or even an original faulty design—a wrongly threaded screw, a metal wire with a gauge far too weak to handle the pressure, a motor too highly powered for the delicate pieces it is meant to gyrate. Sometimes, even, a surprising void, essentials absent from the beginning.

114.

The attorney hands out copies of the signed settlement, then slides across the table two warmed cookies from the café on the ground floor. "I imagine you like chocolate," she says. Between the office and elevators I consume mine, three bites and gone, my fingers squeezing the empty bag, a remaining dark morsel squishing warm between waxed paper folds. His cookie he tucks into his shirt pocket to be saved for later when he will, I know, sit at his desk in the front room of the home we had shared, cold milk in a blue-toned glass, a paper napkin on a plate beside the laptop centered before him, and carefully unwrap the cookie, the chocolate no longer oozing and sticky but firm with an audible crunch.

He walks me to my car. Holds my head to his chest, my tears soaking his shirt. Says, "What is it?" Then the strangest thing: "Listen, you know where to find me, baby."

In the morning the woman I love lies next to me, a wool cap pulled over her head and ears. An impenetrable spiritual core allows Lyn the belief she—a miraculous assembly of moving parts—can be fixed. The word *prognosis* is gone from her vocabulary; she insists I remove it from mine.

A gray mist blankets the beach cottage. Rain taps the roof. "You look terrible," she says.

115.

The long corridor to the oncologist's office holds six large, cheap prints: puffs of pastel blue and white, portraying, I imagine, a cloudlike, heavenly afterworld.

No! No! No! Give me soil, sea, trees, grass!

116.

Always, we pray over the chemo.
Her hand, then mine, resting on the clear bag.

Bless this, let it heal.

117.

Lyn looks down and the oncologist offers me his eyes, his lifted chin, his otherwise expressionless face. He and Lyn joke. Well, Lyn jokes and he joins in. Dr. Gransdorfer. She affectionately calls him Dr. G. They've laughed about everything from the satisfaction of a really good shit to the banality of the music piped into the reception area. Her cancer numbers have taken an initial plunge. Lyn hoots at the news, the kind of shameless shriek a beer-guzzling Southern boy might vent when his team scores the winning touchdown. Dr. G freezes momentarily, this tall, graying, handsome man with an elevated ego. He is all about image and reputation, but when no one on the floor complains, he allows himself a smile.

118.

David sends the boxed set. Remembering her childhood giggles, Lyn pops one of the tapes into the VCR. "The Marx Brothers! Time to laugh!"

119.

Six months into treatment. In the waiting room a couple walks in. He lumbers through the door first, hulking steps. She follows. Her eyes are bloodshot and moist—not tears, but a condition. Everyone here is pumping toxins.

They sit opposite me and Lyn, dropping into padded chairs simultaneously. He fills his space and half hers. The man grabs a newspaper from a side table. His face hidden behind the sports page, he proclaims into the belly of the room, "Yoo-ee, the Skins pulled it out yesterday!" and continues to rattle off game highlights as if anyone cares, as if that morning when the liver is failing and the lungs are filling, as we wait to see the doc and hear news which will be either horrific or only bad, having dragged ourselves through the week with little sleep and less joy, tallying two CT scans, a 2 a.m. drive to the ER, five hours of chemo, and injections to boost the red cells and the white cells and the bone cells, along with infusions of Percocet, Ativan, and morphine . . . we could possibly have any concern for McNabb and his perfect pass or the fighting Philadelphia Eagles and their staggering defeat.

Lyn holds my hand, her eyes closed, her skin as toneless as the morning's pale fog. She's lost nearly twenty pounds.

A few chairs away a shrunken, bald man sits alone, chin dipping toward his concave chest. He clears his throat. "I was rooting for Philly," he says.

120.

When we are shown into an examination room, we are in surprisingly good spirits. We are buying a house and three weeks from settlement, and are reflecting again on the benefit concert to honor Lyn, the musicians she gigged with over the years who had gathered and sung to her, the female duo that hilariously emceed the evening, the hundreds who had come to listen and donate, all the love.

Dr. G walks in, holding the results of the cancer trackers. "Okay. Now. So your numbers are about the same. Back up. A bit. Yes, a bit. But that's what happens. Don't focus on the numbers. Sometimes the numbers will jump, then level off and step down. Sometimes. So we'll just stick with the same protocol this week. And next. Then we'll do another scan. And we'll see how we'll continue."

He flashes me another of his looks that say *I'm telling her this but I don't really believe it and you shouldn't either.*

"Okay," Lyn says. "I just thought I'd be better by now."

121.

"This sucks," she says, "this really sucks."

She wails, beginning slowly at first.
I wrap my arms around her and wail, too.

122.

In step with Lyn's decline comes a surge in libido of those around us. Chris, in a neighboring cottage and alone for years, suddenly finds romance. Her seismic, shrieking orgasms nightly between 1 and 2 a.m. stupefy the neighborhood. When Andy joins us afternoons for coffee on the small front patio, his new girl never fails to phone and he never fails to coo sugar back, though the two just left each other a half hour before. In another nearby cottage, a woman forever trying to lose weight and change her attitude does exactly just that. She drops fifteen pounds and departs daily at dawn for an ocean swim. Apparently she has found a gorgeous fish to keep her company. She waves cheerily outside the screen door, sweat plastering her bangs to her forehead. "Hey, y'all!" she sings to me and Lyn sitting in a darkened room, blinds drawn against the too-bright sun, Lyn sipping bitter tea to cool the inflamed liver. "God, what a bea-u-ti-ful day, isn't it?" She presses her nose briefly to the screen before she flits off.

123.

We searched for a home for more than a year. The first we fell for, the one before the cancer, had an extra room ideal for a recording studio, and an artistically terraced rear yard—like those I'd known in Italy—where we could host intimate salons with poetry and music and friends and guests and round tables dressed in white. The front door was even painted Lyn's favorite bright blue. This perfect house was the one the geologist told us the morning we were officially to sign that it was slipping, yes slipping, see those cracks in the side steps? See how the soil has jumped the curb, is approaching from across the street? It sits on unsteady ground and will slide into the ravine, he said, maybe tomorrow, maybe in a few years, maybe a few more, but it will happen.

The second house, Lyn by then months into treatment, was a postcard cottage two blocks from the beach with a rose garden, a kitchen filled with white marble and sun, room for one grand piano (though not two), and a perfect lower-level apartment with private entry for my son. The day before signing, our friend George offered to inspect the inspector's approval. He found the house had mold. Rotting from the inside out. He pointed to the patched, discolored stucco: irrefutable evidence. His mournful expression said only: You can't buy this house.

The third house is too large, too much ground to maintain, further from town. Still, we pack her things, my things, the two pianos, the cat. We bring them all to the house on the hill, the house of light, the one we finally close on and will for the first time be sharing. Seven days before my fiftieth birthday, Lyn in the dregs of chemo, I hold the keys and sit alone on the deck high above the wide pacific blue and wonder, *What have I done? What will become of my life?*

124.

In May, I plant tomato seedlings beneath an empty moon. *I love you I love you*, I sing to them, a mini prayer. I stab a couple tiny sticks into the ground, crutches to keep them upright. *I need you to live.*

125.

A friend offers to take Lyn to an appointment. "Get some air, some sun!" she tells me. "You look dreadful." Size 4 jeans fall from my hips. My once honeyed skin is ghastly pale. Between my brows: the beginning of a serious, irreversible fold.

I open all the windows, *the house to myself.* Outside, a plane pulls through a heavy palette of gray, cuts the sky in half. A thin, white scar floating there, still, when they return.

126.

Robert, come to tune our pianos, is shaking his head, his face ashen at the news of Lyn's diagnosis. "I've got to sit," he wheezes, hand on heart, though he's already parked on my couch.

His face questions. "She's away at treatment," I say.

"You know," he turns to me, his thinly woven dress shirt ready to spring buttons, his hair thinning and greased, a Bluetooth light at his ear, "You know how there's a term for women who hang around gay men?" I nod. "Fag hag," he says anyway and adds a disparaging wiggle of his hand.

"Well," he says, "well, I'm the male equivalent . . . and they just don't have a word for my type. [*Dyke dick* was Lyn's favorite phrase.] I've always loved lesbians," he says. "Sassy and self-assured. And Lynda . . . God, I've been in love with her ever since I can remember."

I show him to the large front room where Lyn's Baldwin now rests, the room planned to become her recording studio when she was better, when she felt like playing and composing again.

Robert gets to work, taming harsh flats and sharps, gradually returning the piano to perfect concert pitch. Minutes later, a prolonged quiet. I find him sitting at her piano, fingers stroking the keys, his face puckered and damp.

"Geez," he says and leaves.

127.

We exhaust eight full seasons of *The West Wing*, all seasons of *Doc Martin*, *Downton Abbey*, *Sherlock*, and a number of French and Italian films. Lyn swallows her benzo drugs, holding off until 4 p.m. so they'll last her through the evening. *Hardball* from 4 to 5, *Frasier* from 5 to 6 or 7, then PBS news, then *Two and a Half Men*.

One evening after watching the movie *Julie and Julia*, we find the real Julia Child, a staple of both our childhoods. "Episode 1: Boeuf Bourguignon." My MacBook settled on a small square pillow on the bed, speaker plugged into the side. Lyn holds my hand, tries not to feel nauseous. Other than salami with lots of fat, she hasn't eaten meat for months.

128.

My grandmother, on her returns from visiting family in Italy, smuggled through U.S. Customs rolls of fresh salami shoved up the sleeves of her heavy woolen coat. Her brothers made the salami themselves; there was nothing in America to compare.

When the customs officers asked if she had any farm meat products, she'd shake her head, "No, no," and walk by.

What was she doing wrong? she'd insist later. Rules, she taught, were open to interpretation. Good intentions entitled you to a pass.

129.

I think every woman should have a blowtorch.

Julia Child

130.

"Would you like a soft egg?"

"You know what I'd really like?" she says. "Your potatoes."

I put potatoes on to boil, return, and hand her a glutamine drink, her medications.

"*Fried* potatoes, right?"

I remove the parboiled potatoes from the water, slice them into butter, and turn the heat up to crisp. I sit with her again.

"With feta?"

I stir the potatoes, put feta on them, bring her the plate.

"You know what else?" she says. "Cornichons."

131.

Later she needs the oxygen turned on, and could I bring her a grape Gatorade, and get her pain medication?

I say yes. And again yes. And always yes.

132.

My foot lands in a sticky Gatorade blot on the wood floor. When Lyn dozes, I take a damp cloth to the Rorschach. Purple flares shoot outward from a steady center, tendrils reaching, reaching.

A swipe of the cloth, and the remaining drops crawl out again.

133.

Strangely, I think of you then, though I can't remember when you first claimed the bottom of my childhood bed or how many months you terrorized me there, your coiled serpent body pulsating, your grotesque head rising the moment I shut off the light.

I'd search in the closet, behind the dresser, under the box spring, assuring myself that I was alone in the room. Yet even as I lay awake, darkness brought your certain return.

I learned the ancient Greeks regarded you as sacred and wise. When curled around a staff, you become a symbol of healing. Oh, but how you haunted me. Your ominous stare seizing my throat.

When I told Laura about you, she said, "He's still there in your subconscious. Find him. Confront him. *What was it he wanted?*"

134.

. . . We always had this theory that if you saw—if you kept the snake in your eye line, the snake wasn't going to bite you. And that's kind of the way I feel about confronting pain. I want to know where it is.

Joan Didion, *NPR interview 2005*

135.

Our evening routine, the TV on. Lyn reclines on the sofa, legs stretched across my lap. It's *Frasier* time. Thirty seconds in, I realize I know this one. It's a rerun of a rerun. The sitcom had eleven seasons, each season with twenty-four episodes. Two hundred sixty-four shows total. At five reruns per week, it comes to fifty-two weeks' worth. Exactly one year, which seems about right. We've now viewed them all.

I consider hunting for a pack of playing cards, hoping for a diversion, but I've forgotten the games I once knew, can only conjure up War, that fast and witless homage to dull chance. The victor holding all the cards in the end.

136.

My grandfather handed me the deck. I cut the cards once, twice, three times just to be sure. A chilled bottle of Michelob sweated on the linoleum table between us. He poured a splash into a small glass and slid it my way. I was ten. He would die in a year from bad lungs, though neither of us knew this then.

He'd find a way to cheat—steal an extra card, disappear one under his palm. Then slyly he'd let on that he did, knowing I'd shout—Poppi!—throw down my cards, and stomp off.

This was the game, his game. My fiery response the cherished moment he waited for. Maybe it was the promise that his granddaughter would one day be a woman with spirit.

La mia bellissima! he called after me, laughing.

137.

My mother, his daughter, would later sadly observe me, and I imagined she was asking herself what she had several times asked me directly: Where is my Lisa? Where has she gone? For she, too, had lost something of herself in marriage. *"What has happened to you?"* I overheard a longtime friend say to her.

138.

"Leave him," my mother had said. "Come home with the kids. Dad will help." It was that last move that convinced her. He'd flown ahead with a suitcase as he'd done in the past, and I packed our belongings one more time, said all the goodbyes. I tried to explain his shocking insistence to return to California—uprooting the kids again after just nine months in their new happy home back East, near my mother, already seriously ill, and my father, my sisters—but there was no explaining this one.

139.

I balance atop an eight-foot ladder in the skylight alcove by the front door, a quart of paint clasped in one hand, a wide brush in the other.

"Red?" Lyn is unconvinced.

I dip the brush and quickly slather crimson over the white—thick, sloppy strokes—hearing my father softly admonish, "One thin coat, Lisa, a thin coat, let it dry, then another," a method I'd always followed, until now. There is nowhere to go, no plans for the remainder of the day, yet there is this urgency.

The goal is warmth and the result is immediate: a luminous glow singing in.

140.

Once, sometimes twice, each week we enter the hospital lobby and wait. Lyn riding in the portable wheelchair, I steering from behind. Each time, the same cheery instructions, the same thick stack of admission papers to initial and sign, the same plastic hospital band to be snipped off and tossed hours later. Lyn is unfailingly gracious and patient, thanking the clerk, asking how their day is going. The clerk is unfailingly delighted at the attention, and feeling at ease, turns to me, curious.

Don't ask me if I am her friend.
Don't ask me if I am her sister.
Don't ask me if I am her daughter.
Do that one more time and *I will destroy you.*

I am her partner, her lover, the one she was to grow old with.
No, you have no idea.

141.

Deep in meditation, she leans into the pain, her body draped over a metal cart, the first long needle inserted to numb what it can, the second puncturing the flesh of her back and the swollen lung sac, pleural fluid fleeing through a tube into a pouch, sometimes a liter, sometimes more, pale yellow in color with an occasional worrisome tint.

No one knows whether it is the cancer or the chemotherapy that is determined to drown her.

142.

Dr. G's answer to Lyn's request for a scrip for medicinal pot: No. Legal here in California, but not nationwide. No, he won't do it. OxyContin, Percocet, Valium: not a problem. But no scrip for a joint. He is determined to keep his stellar reputation alive. "I'm quite certain," he says with a despicable nod, "that with your . . . friends . . . you can acquire some on your own."

143.

I drop the car windows a couple inches to let in the day, its warmth. The sun's breeze blows through my hair, strands flap against my face.

"Darling," Lyn says, powering her window back up, "it's so fucking cold."

144.

One day, another day, and another. Another week. Another month.

145.

The *Take one!* box in the treatment center overflows with knitted caps in olive and tangerine. Lyn wears a similar cap in navy and lavender, last season's shades. Her thick blond curls gave up and dropped away in clumps sometime last year.

"How's it going?" Lyn calls to Brad and Anna, nurses who have become extended family. Brad, in his cheery plum fatigues, is solemn, his usual "Hey, Lynda!" absent. Anna smiles, forgoes her generous hug.

The further they pull away, the closer the end, a nurse friend told me months ago. They've been slowly killing her. Dr. G is ultimately responsible, but they injected the poison toxic enough to dissolve skin on contact. The treatments are not helping and there is no turning back.

146.

Lyn and I, too, are pulling away. From music. From poetry. From what drew us together, brought us joy. Our relationship is beginning to feel like an ongoing end with no beginning. No, that isn't right. It had a sensually explosive beginning. It is the entire middle that is missing.

147.

I wrap an arm around her. Her feet shuffle along the sand-toned tweed carpet. Tiny steps, we make our way. Toward the door. Toward home.

Propped at eye level, the booklet displays prominently in front of the others, a new addition to the rack of informational brochures in the waiting room. On its cover: *Sex and Cancer*, in pastel script, and below, two faces. A mature man and woman, gray hair neatly combed, skin a perky peach tint, their profiles approaching for a tight-lipped kiss.

I stare at the cover's sanitized image. Cancer is messy. So is sex when it's good. Where is the heat, the hunger? What about the still-young, what about the gay men and women, what about lovers just beginning whose lives have been kicked over and spilt out?

148.

You want to design a brochure about sex and cancer? Put on its cover a woman in her prime, luminescent eyes beneath missing brows, face tilted back. Her expression is complex: the memory of ecstasy, the craving to feel its surge again. To be able to again. Her lover sits next to her on an unmade bed. The lover's lips are buried in the woman's pale neck. You can't see the tears but you know they are there.

149.

And inside, this is what you write:

There are three of you now, cancer present in every touch. Be vigilant. Hold each moment. Gather them. For however uncomfortable sex is now, the next time will be more so. Prepare yourself. *Understand, there will be a last time.* And you will know it. In the breath immediately following, you will know it.

Later there will come the second death, the full-body one. Then, there will be others around, to whisper yes, to witness. Then, you will be held.

But there will first be this. And this death you will bear alone.

150.

Lyn clutches a hand-sized velvet heart filled with lavender pearls, LOVE etched in fine white across its belly.

She whispers, *My body is healing, love will beat this.*

151.

"Your heart is strong," he tells her, the chipper, fresh-faced nurse, tanned and muscular with a mop of blond curls. He holds the results of the echocardiogram ordered when, after eighteen months of chemo, Lyn felt something was seriously off. "No worries, it'll be pumping when you're ninety!" His white grin is almost neon.

Lyn doesn't know: My heart is compromised. One of the valves pumps oddly—potentially in the wrong direction—causing the other three to work more than their share. "Worry will only increase its stress," I was told at the time of the test, some eight years ago. "It's managed until now. No reason to believe it won't keep on. . . ." A stroke, was my cardiologist's reasoning. Something in the past. Likely a traumatic event. "I don't recall," I said. "With a shock of that intensity, I'd be surprised if you did," he said.

In the car, she takes the seat belt strap from me when I try to help. "I'm good, baby." After five attempts, it snaps in. We back out of the hospital lot. A gaunt hand drops to my thigh. She is still smiling. "What a relief," she says.

152.

The chicken, washed and dried, splays on the cutting board. With a sharp knife, I sever the legs from the carcass, carve away the breasts. The meat saved for later dinners, the bones and wings for broth.

I reach inside the damp cavity and extract liver, gizzard, heart. Sautéed and spooned over toast, the organs are her current wish. I slice the gizzard wafer thin, slide it into the hot skillet. A diced shallot, two smashed tears of garlic. Salt, more salt. A spoon of butter. Salt for flavor, fat to ease the passage. *No parsley, darling. Tastes like paper, I can't get it down.*

Next, the liver. Vein removed, coarsely chopped, tossed in. A single stir and the aroma blooms. I turn down the heat. In the next room, the oxygen machine spits a monotonous, metallic wheeze. Oomph-zahhhhhhh. Oomph-zahhhhhhh. On and on and on, the din surrounding my mother as she lay dying from the same sick lungs. I dial the fan to high and hide my face over the skillet.

The tender heart waits. I cut it in half and drop it in.

153.

Yes, we're certain.
No, there is no mistake.

No, no mistake.

154.

Midnight. I slouch on a metal stool under biting hospital lights, praying. The emergency medical staff is trying to revive Lyn. It came on suddenly, a slurring of words, babbling nonsense, her muscles weakening, within a half hour a near loss of consciousness. My sister, who'd spent the week with us, had left hours before. I call her at the airport. She skips her redeye east and drives back to be at my side.

But it doesn't happen. Not that night. In the morning Lyn sits up and scrutinizes our weary faces, says, "What the hell was that all about?"

Days later we know the cause. She mistook her Ativan—a benzodiazepine for anxiety—for another prescription. Swallowed nine tiny pills of it. The doc is relieved the mystery is solved, but incredulous, repeating into the phone—you can almost hear him shaking his head—*How did you . . . the odds against surviving that. . . .*

155.

Andy lets himself in and settles into a chair in the darkened bedroom, on watch, freeing me for a walk in the light. I am about to leave the room when Lyn wakens and steps from the bed, nude, and wobbles to the bathroom, crossing Andy's path. She doesn't see him, her eyes half shut, her focus a direct line to the bathroom and back. But he sees her. The fright on his face. My despair at witnessing it. If she still had muscle—her authentic body-building self—they both would have enjoyed the surprise. But hers is a body on the verge of giving way, a reality so crushingly private, no one, not even Andy, has the right.

156.

Every Breath is Healing

A cloth scroll. It arrives in the mail, another gift from David. I pin it vertically inside by the front door.

157.

She can't remember. Not how the Logic Pro program works, how one exports a midi file, how to get the Mac to play the orchestrated pieces she composed. She can't even remember Tom's name, the musician she's been working with closely, has known for years. "Mike?" she says. "Is that it?"

Several secondary schools and a university had taken an interest in her musical compositions and had featured them in their lessons. The choral-orchestral project was to be her legacy; it required finally only a couple intense pushes to bring it into the world. But then the cancer came and everything stopped.

158.

There are challenges which, although at first appear to be complex, can be made quite simple if viewed from a different perspective. Adding the numbers from one to ten, for example. The answer is immediate and refreshingly clear when you write them out and realize that the numbers are actually five groups of eleven: 1 and 10, 2 and 9, 3 and 8, 4 and. . . .

And then there are those problems—say, a progression of events—which no matter how you analyze them or group them, remain fucked with no possibility of simplification.

159.

"It will be difficult, Lisa," he tells me, taking me aside, this close friend of Lyn's family, another famed doctor, when he comes to visit. "Very difficult. Soon." His expression is grave. His solemn nod assures he speaks the truth. I want to ask what he means by that, by "very difficult," for I can't imagine anything worse than what now is, but he is already back with Lyn, his elegantly suited body sitting beside her too-thin one, his strong hands sandwiching hers.

160.

My once-husband, his new wife, and I sit in Berkeley's stadium bleachers at a perilous height. Our daughter is somewhere far below, standing in a queue which winds from the 50-yard line graduation podium, down the length of the football field, along a sidewalk, across Bancroft and Durant, then onward still, she, one of several thousand, waiting for her moment.

Four years ago, she and I drove here for the first time, the family van filled to bursting. Lyn had flown up then to be with us, to help settle her into her new home, to share the long return drive with me.

From around the stadium, continued bursts of celebratory cheers. The clouds have suddenly burned off, the morning's gray chill gone. Below us, a family opens an umbrella against the sun. "It's too hot," the man I have shared my life with says. He clomps down metal stairs aiming for a square of shade by the goalposts at the end of the field, his wool sweater left draped over the metal beside me. His wife stands and follows. A guard approaches them, there is some discussion, and they walk off.

He maybe has been the father he could be, I reason. He's proud of his children, provided for them. He'd grown up in a family struggling emotionally and economically in a country rebuilding from a world war it had begun and lost. The American hoopla over life events is something he never understood.

And yet. Today is undeniably momentous. A *commencement*, a beginning. An event worthy of reflection, a moment of joy.

My cell rings. "This is so difficult," Sam begins, his words rushing out. He's at our home, caring for his sister the few days I am here. Lyn was thrilled to see him when he arrived—it had been months—still, she didn't want me to leave. Nor did Sam, acutely shaken by her physical decline. "I mean Lynnie's not with it." I hear the fear. I understand, but I cannot help him now. "The nurse tried to show me the morphine, I couldn't listen, even look. I mean . . . *When will you be back?*"

I slip from my sandals; sunbaked metal scorches my feet. "Day after tomorrow." He knows this.

Nearing the stage, she is radiant. Her graceful stance, the way she turns her head—I would spot her if she were another hundred yards away. "Mom!" she texts. She looks in my direction though she has no idea where I sit. I jump up. Water bottles careen off the bleacher.

161.

Be here now, a piano instructor wrote long ago on a Bach suite, his letters upright, bold. It was a command, not a suggestion: Be present, or give it up.

162.

Sam flies home to New York the day I return, and now, two weeks later, it is David who will stay with Lyn while I leave for three days to be with family in Baltimore, my uncle's eightieth birthday party. David insists I go, to "hopefully laugh a little." I am withering, and he sees it.

"Lynda was the first one I came out to as a teen," David says, "and she was there for me when my partner died." He loves her. And in the time I've known him, he's come to love me, too.

"I've got broth on the stove, chicken livers in the oven," David tells me over the phone when I land in Maryland. "But she's not doing well, Lisa. I gave her a bit of morphine this afternoon. She said she wanted to be knocked out entirely. I told her you were coming back. She needed to stay awake for you."

163.

"Oh, my love." She shivers. Two down blankets and still there's no calming her.

A finger glides along my chin. "I can't give you what you need. Go find it, get it, wherever, whoever: woman . . . [pause] . . . man . . . [a smile]. Just take care of yourself."

164.

"Always go for *the music*," she told me early on. "The notes are much less important."

165.

The rose plucked from our garden and placed by her bedside murmurs from the glass vase, an urgent plea. In the morning, wasted petals lie puddled on the table, sputtered on the floor, too delicate to withstand the chemicals fleeing Lyn's skin throughout the night.

At the open window, a mockingbird stirs. *See me hear me love me!* he squawks, offering up all he has, a clamorous melody patchwork, unable to settle on a voice, not knowing which tenor might reach his mate.

166.

I sing to her softly. Her words, her music.

I tell myself, careful, you don't want to wake her.
But this is not the truth. *I only want to wake her,*
shake her from this disease, take her from this hideous tomb.

I place her hand on the warm soft of my belly; my skin quivers.

I miss you, baby.

Outside, a pale, celestial light.
Dawn. One more. But one more means one less.

167.

Unable to sleep, I scan the titles of Lyn's books pressed into the bedside cabinet. A shelf of novels: Isabel Allende, Gore Vidal, Barry Unsworth, Susan Sontag. Another of inquisitive, philosophical reads: *The Gnostic Gospels*, *The Duino Elegies*, *Man and His Symbols*, *Art and Fear*, *Team of Rivals*.

I reach over and lift out *Care of the Soul*. A bookmark slips out.

Angels can fly, it advises in a pale, feathery blue,
because they take themselves so lightly.

168.

"Are they real?" my young niece asked. She held a doll-sized angel in her arms, white gown, stuffed silver wings. "Have you seen one?"

"Yes," I said. "More than one. But they weren't dressed in white, and if they had wings, they were tucked away."

"How did you know, then?"

"Because they did what angels do: show up unexpectedly when you need help. Angels stand suddenly before you, extend their hand in greeting, and offer what they can—and it is quite a lot. And then! When you turn away and look back, they are gone."

169.

Adoria, hospice nurse, stands before me with two hot teas, one for her, one for me, everything aligned on a tray—spoons, my sugar decanter, a dish with sweets, a separate small plate for the used tea bags—her eyes bulging as if they might pop, her face lost in teased-out blond hair. (Lyn's friend Sid, who's driven an hour every day this week after work to be here with Lyn, with me, her love absolute, pulled me aside when she first met Adoria. "That one's family," she said approvingly. Lesbian.)

I haven't seen that small plate in years. Where did she find it? How much rummaging did she do in my kitchen to uncover it? I have to admit, though, it is a perfect size, a proper complement to the teacup and saucer, the glass dish with the chocolates and Torrone nougat she found in the pantry.

They have been omnipresent, the hospice nurses, administering meds and making critical decisions, journaling Lyn's condition drug by drug, heartbeat by heartbeat. In their presence I feel powerless, a spectator adrift with nothing to define the hours.

"No, thank you," I say. Adoria nods and looks away, and for one brief moment, I have the upper hand.

170.

Every five minutes: *Lynda, this is your nurse Adoria. I'm going to give you your medication now.* Drops under her tongue. Again and again and again: *Lynda, this is your nurse Adoria. I'm going to give you your medication now.*

Six of us hushed on the bed, helpless, holding on. Lyn, me, Andy, Eve, Sid, and Ellen, a new and cherished friend. When Adoria steps away briefly, Sid says sotto voce: *Adoria, this is Lynda's lawyer Sid. I'm going to . . . sue the fuck out of you if you say that one more time.*

And we in our huddle softly laugh, a crazed desperation, knowing Lyn would have appreciated the wry humor, laughed along, if she weren't almost gone.

171.

The smell of roasting vegetables wafts into the bedroom. A complex, shocking aroma. Someone is cooking in our kitchen. A figure (who?) stands at the door. Looks in. Turns away.

A darkening window. An intense quiet in this room where so much has happened. Life stripped, fading. Eve and Ellen curl at the bottom. Andy stretches near me, his hand gentle on my leg, my hand over Lyn's heart, watching her face, whispering to her. And Sid, sitting behind Lyn, supporting her, when she dies.

172.

The next morning I find the hospice's blue binder, mistakenly left behind, pages upon pages of dated entries. The last lines are Adoria's.

Her swirling black ink.   Then emptiness.   And then this:

8:15 PT expired.

173.

My Love,

After your spirit flew, I somehow made my way up the stairs and found myself outside—as if you were pulling me. In the still evening quiet, I sat alone on the curb. The mortuary arrived. I may have said something. Or not. I remember two or three people, carrying your body away. Then just in front of me, hidden in a tree, a mama owl called *whoo-whoo . . . whoo*, followed by a baby's hesitant *whoo.* Again and again the mama sang out, celebrating the new life, the just-born responding with a single, wondrous *whoo*, watching the house, watching me. A rustle of feathers. They waited. "Okay," I said. "Okay." (How could there still be tears?) Then the mama once more, and the baby once more, and then they flew. And there was only the warm breeze, the black-blue heaven, the stars beginning to light.

174.

I call Dr. G's office to cancel the appointment. Five rings, then a chipper voice followed by a long beep. "Lynda died," I say, phone at my ear, listening, until the recorder clicks off.

No one calls back.

175.

Lyn's sister phones from Israel, where she's lived for some forty years. "Oh, Lisa. . . ." I know her own cancer has returned.

She asks if I can find out the exact time the cremation will take place. She wants to be reciting a special Hebrew prayer as her sister's body becomes ash. A wish so profound, it makes me weep.

176.

My son, on summer college break, drives the fifty minutes from his father's.

We sit quietly awhile.
"Hungry?" I say.

In the kitchen, we open the pantry, pull from shelves wide noodles, onions, garlic, tomato puree. From the fridge: cheeses and cream, broth and carrots. From the front garden: zucchini, basil, oregano. And we begin, side by side, dicing, slicing, stirring. Preparing lasagna. Building it layer by layer.

177.

Lyn's sixtieth birthday. Missed by six days. In a café, hanging near the pastry counter, staring back at me, a six-foot vintage poster, Les Couronnes Sodas Limonades: a human-size clown smothered in white fluff, a soda bottle balanced on his pale forehead. The amped music—a mix of The Stones, Willie Nelson, Frank Sinatra, and Kool and the Gang—turns to Carol King's "It's Too Late," a song Lyn performed for her first band audition all those years ago, a song she sang for me.

I get the call. Eve picks me up. Together we drive to the mortuary. Inside, an attendant waits: thin frame draped in black, manly fedora pressed onto her raven hair. The place reeks of pathos, dust. Ahead a hallway ends in darkness. She leads us into a small side room. We don't sit. An anemic finger slides the container of Lyn's remains across the roughhewn surface of her desk. "Sign and you can go," she says.

"*Can you imagine, can you?*" I say to Eve as we stand stunned in the parking lot. "Lyn being there these past days? In that hell?"

178.

"I'm sorry, baby," is all I can think to say as I cradle the small canister of her ashes in my arms. I'm sorry.

179.

My daughter, traveling in Asia with friends, sobs when I tell her. "I'll come home, Mama!"

"No, no . . . I'll see you soon."

180.

Johanna Solis leaves a voice message on the landline. "Hi, Lynda. We have our weekly appointment scheduled for this time. I'll check my voice messages to see if you left me something."

Johanna performed healings over the phone, at an impressive cost. She insisted that she could see Lyn's cells, could target the ones actually dividing—the ravenous, bestial, cancerous ones—and annihilate them. Lyn's spiritual nature allowed her to accept Johanna's promise at first. As the months wore on, Lyn felt only shittier, though she continued the sessions: If she were to stop believing in the power to heal, then what?

Again a half hour later. "Hi, this is Johanna Solis. I realize you might not be able to come to the phone, I'll just begin my work. . . ."

I pick up. "Hello, Johanna, this is Lisa."

"Oh, Lisa!"

"Lynda died this past Saturday."

"Oh . . . Oh . . . I didn't know. . . ." *How did you not know?* "Well, what I can do is say a prayer to get her to a good place in her new life." *Go to hell, Johanna.* "I'm so sorry, Lisa, so sorry. I know how you cared for her these past months." *Do you?* "Goodbye, Lisa. God bless."

181.

The memorial is outdoors, on a cliff above the ocean. A rabbi,
a gathering of friends, two of Lyn's cousins and their families.
My sister, her daughter, my son at my side.

Lyn's longtime soulmate, Karen, singing, reminiscing.
A squadron of pelicans swooping overhead.

I do what I can. There is nothing, nothing left.

182.

The condolences, the phone messages. Men, distraught, weeping. They can't believe the news. They knew Lynda, or had known her some years ago, or had maybe once spoken to her. "She was . . ." they begin, unable to finish.

183.

In Lyn's drawer the day she died, June 2, 2012:

Lactase
Dairy Ease
Hydromorphone
Dilaudid
Trazodone
Rhubarb root
Slippery elm bark
Prochlorperazine
Pantoprazole
Betaine HCL Pepsin
Darvocet
Oxycodone
Burdock root
Sheep sorrel
Wheat germ
Coriolus
Lipoic acid
L-Carnitine
L-Ornithine
Melatonin
Hycodan
Protonix

Warfarin
Fentanyl
Lovenox
Roxicet
Medrol
Zofran
Ativan
Norco

184.

I show a friend the contents of the drawer.

"If that stuff finds its way into the ocean, the fish are fucked," she says.

185.

When Lyn entered hospice, a chaplain called the house, asked if he could help out, was Lynda interested in confession, preparing for her passage with Jesus? "She's Jewish," I said, "we're good." And besides, I wanted to add, *she's not dying.*

Weeks later I sit with another eight mourners gathered around an oval table in the Sunshine Room, the same chaplain presiding. Seven stacks of cards fill the table's center, each a shade, the chaplain explains, representing a stage of grief. Shock/denial is first in the line, a bright red. Choose one, he says. Where are we in this moment?

I look at the woman sitting to my right, her uncombed nest of wild curls, openly sobbing, furiously working through a box of tissues. A withered man to my left is a mournful slump in his chair. I stand, reach over the table, and select white. Acceptance.

"What is it you miss?" the chaplain wants to know.
I imagine myself asking: How honest may I be?

Then suddenly, there is this: The rattle of ice in her glass of Scotch. That jingle, just before the sip.

186.

A sheet of linen cardstock, pale soft white, a soothing hue.
Its purity watches from the surface of my desk.

I position the pen center page. Black ink glides over ivory.
Three syllables, five, then again three.

My dearest,

It is so quiet

without you.

187.

My daughter spends the remainder of the summer with me. "Mom," she says, "maybe you can begin clearing out that room." The room once imagined to become a recording studio.

"It's best," I say.

"You can do Craigslist. For that huge sofa. We'll take a photo, say—gotta be honest—'Down cushions, top-grade butterscotch leather. Worn. Some cat claw damage. Perfect fraternity couch.' You'll see, someone will call and haul it out of here within an hour."

She is really trying. I am trying, too.

188.

The piano movers call to arrange transport of Lyn's piano to New York. Though Sam is unable to read music, he plays well by ear. It is his now, this instrument that produced the astonishing tones that had inspired and soothed her. Its keys knew her touch for fifty years.

"Sam," I say to him on the phone. "Sam, she's left you the Baldwin."

"Really?" Then moments of silence. His voice falls: "Where am I going to put it?"

189.

I call the piano guy back. "I'll be there Monday," he says, "to have a look. My crew will arrive Tuesday to haul it out."

"No," I say. "No, not Tuesday." Why is there no air? "I won't be ready," I insist. "Maybe later, next week."

190.

I sit in my courtyard with Dan, an engaging, eccentric engineer, graying, lanky. Between us, a plate of Madeleines, whipped cream, and chocolates. He sweeps a Madeleine through the cream and swallows without tasting. "You and Lynda," he says. "Your electricity, your radiation: It matched." He pauses. "It was honestly beautiful to watch." He eyes a Ghirardelli square, then lifts it on edge between forefinger and thumb. He is thinking, I think, that the chocolate is not quite square, not square at all, off by a fractional millimeter or so, when he turns to me and says, "Such a thing is a rarity. But you had it, Lisa. You had it."

Who can say why Lyn—a brilliant, sensual being—was taken in the prime of her creativity? Dan points to two lemon trees in my garden, one infested with a pestilence which deforms its leaves, curling them yellow, though the branches are heavy with tasty, ripened fruit. The neighboring tree is green and tall, seemingly stronger, but almost barren of sweetness. "It's a crapshoot," he says.

191.

Lyn's boxes which she'd kept sealed shut in the garage are walled around me, now open, her life scattered across the floor. Girl band photos from the '70s, '80s, from gigs in LA, in Vegas, in Atlantic City, in Monte Carlo, in New York, at Carnegie Hall. At a concert grand. In a sports coupe puffing a badass stogie. At her commitment ceremony to the golf star. Reel-to-reel tapes. Her CDs. Her written music, the original notated compositions, including the songs she composed for me.

Dan, back again to repair my garden wall, comes in for a drink and finds me sprawled on the rug. His brilliant mind long ago determined (with proof, he assures) that life as we know it is an illusion. He nods, considers commenting. Doesn't. He walks to the kitchen and returns with his sippy cup refilled. "Lisa," the gravity of his voice acknowledging my ravaged face, "it may be too soon."

192.

I tell Dan of my last moments with Lyn. How she was holding on with inhuman strength. How I lay next to her in our bed, surrounded by friends. How I tapped a strength I didn't know *I* had, whispering to her again and again, a mantra almost, "Baby, you can let go now. I love you. I will be okay. Let go. Go to sleep. I love you so." How maybe more than the words, it was my hand above her heart, the slow circular motion my fingers felt compelled to make, that let her understand.

Dan listens, visibly touched. "You should know," he says, "it's been proven—1982, to be exact—that two quantum particles once connected, then separated by the vastest of distances, *remain connected.* Continue in some form to interact. Exactly how is still uncertain. [He shrugs.] Mind-blowing. And true."

193.

On hangers, in drawers, folded on shelves: Lyn's clothes fill half the closet still, weeks later. The softest sweaters, the destroyed tees, her favorite red plaid flannel shirt I will save for myself. But what with the rest? I consider asking Eve to come by, have a look. But thinking of her scrutinizing Lyn's wardrobe, buttoning on her linen blouses, tugging the jackets to see how they might fit . . . I can't bear it.

I sit on the floor, her shoes at my side: Ferragamo pumps in burgundy and coal, leather boots, cross-trainers. I turn and a sleeve of a silk blouse, a favorite of her evening gigs, brushes my chin.

194.

Family members call, ask what I'm doing. I say *nothing much*, when I'm honest. *But you must do something!* they insist, their voices elevating to a worried squeal. *Action is good!* They cannot know, cannot see, that inside I'm being carved out at an incredible rate.

I am widow! I want to bellow, holding the word up as a shield. *Widow*, I want to declare. *Empty*.

195.

A small table, a cool beer. A local blues band.
"We're having a good time," I say in a phone message to David.
Though he knows Lyn died a month ago. Though I sit here, alone.

196.

Can you imagine, can you?

197.

With my daughter in New York, hunting for her new home, we exit the hotel elevator. Eva Cassidy's "Fields of Gold" falls from speakers, swarms the lobby. Lyn's song. Lyn singing! I sprint for the entrance. It's been only six weeks.

"Mom! What are you doing, Mom, wait!"

198.

In a large, unmarked box in the garage I find some fifty black-and-white scholastic notebooks. Her journals. I lift out a few, each cover clearly dated in her unmistakable script. The most recent appears to be from June 2010, just prior to the diagnosis, more than two years ago. I take out several more, searching for one chronicling the months of our beginning, which was when, really? When we first kissed? First made love? First thought about a life together? I choose one from 2007. Toy with putting it back. I open it.

The words are heartbreaking: concerns over my marriage, that I was still (too) deeply tied to my old life, to my children. Her remarkable, unflinching love for me. She openly voiced all this while alive. What devastates is the full depth of her despair, that our relationship might never actually *be.*

Each daily entry, I notice, closes with the same phrase:
Keep me open to accept the way forward.

I reseal the lid with a fresh strip of tape. What should I do with it? Burn it, I hear her say.

199.

. . . It's all right for parents to rifle through a daughter's
bedroom cabinets to uncover her intimate life,
because they must know, and if she doesn't confide
in them, how else will they find out?
And when her journal—a black hardbound with
PRIVATE red-stenciled across the cover
and wrapped twice around with rubber band—
is, upon arrival at summer camp, unpacked
from her duffel, her mother taps it and says,
"You don't want this lying around where anyone
can pick it up, do you? Let me take it back with me.
I'll put it in your room."

You hand it over, your faith as pure
as the innocuous entries in the book;
it's not until your parents' car disappears
beyond the trees that there is a sinking Oh!

200.

The eight in the Sunshine Room nod in agreement: It is the number of years spent together that make a loss so profound. I understand, or think I can. I left my husband of twenty-four years, the man I at twenty-three fell for, packed my life in a suitcase and moved around the world with, had two children with. The mournfulness almost more painful than with death, because it was an end by choice, an agonizing, harrowing decision. But I know, too, about the ending of a different kind of love, a deeply honest one, suddenly, miraculously there. Surely its destruction is just as cruel?

201.

Sam calls. "It's here. The Baldwin. Arrived yesterday."

"How is it?"

"Incredible. Amazing . . ." Silence. Then a few random chords in a minor key. The beginning of a melody. "Damn, I miss her," he says.

202.

George and I are riding in his Ford truck. Windows down, dry dusty air fills the cab. George is master builder and friend. Thick white hair, hefty mustache. Brought into my life as have so many, through Lyn. We are on our way to a stone yard to find something bold to surround my fireplace. Piled against a fence, we see it: a slab of priceless red, green, and gold onyx, damaged, discarded. There's no one piece large enough for what we need, but there are plenty of pieces. I crouch beside him. "Yes?"

Back home, we spread the stone over the patio. Two chunks quickly pair, but there are still eighteen or so more to consider, some daggers, others near perfect squares. We reassemble what we can, yet everywhere there are small gaps, fragments lost forever.

Our shadows hover over the once masterwork. We consider grinding remnant stone into powder and blending it with clear epoxy for filler. To heal the wounds. But epoxy expands as it dries, potentially resulting in further destruction. Still, we think we must try. There's a chance it may work. And what is the alternative?

203.

It is not until after the water—so much water, ankle deep—
is sucked from the house, the restoration crew come and gone,
the burst pipe repaired, not until after I sit stunned in a
closet and weep

that I realize

nothing of importance has been destroyed—not a photograph,
computer, nor work of art—my piano especially spared, water
encroaching to within inches of its legs, then strangely halting

that I know

she is behind the flood, protecting the sacred while forcing a
cleanse, her fierce love washing away the disease and sadness,
wanting for me a fresh start, insisting on it.

204.

Dan brings a wet vac. Andy drags a sopped carpet into the courtyard. George gathers a crew to restore, rebuild.

205.

Three months later, the house refreshed, I collapse in the room where Lyn's piano once stood, now a bedroom. For days I lie beneath a canopy, blinds drawn against the bright pounding of day, shadows disappearing into the thickness of night. I wonder whether in this darkness the snake might return, if it will finally reveal what it wanted so long ago. Laura had said it would, if I asked, when I was ready.

I am ready.

206.

In the early hours I wake up renewed, lighter.

207.

I know what I am looking for, but locating it among the boxes of wide manila folders—detailed though they are—is a challenge. There is so much here. Lyn's original compositions for the visionary, historical project she began the year we met, and then hadn't the months or years to complete. She's bequeathed it all to me, this breathtaking trove of orchestral and choral harmonies.

I find it—her handwritten score of the Nineteenth Amendment to the Constitution, the decree giving a woman the right to vote, to proffer her views and have them counted.

I will enlarge it, frame it, hang it in the living room. A reminder—a promise.

208.

Midmorning the neighbor's newborn wails *come-get-me!* Next door the trio from hell begin the routine: The dad threatens, the two daughters taunt, all three holler. Car doors slam.

I should be doing something, something *more.* A voice chimes in. "It is time, it is time," it sings. "Yes," I say. "But please: Time for *what*?"

209.

Along the canyon road it slithers toward me, colorfully ornate and longer than I am tall, its progress drunken slow as if it awakened from a long slumber, its skin neon against the black asphalt. I stop and it continues its steady approach, close enough to challenge me if it were to choose, then slips off the edge of the road into the chaparral and is gone.

210.

I locate the Brahms collection, open it to Lyn's inscription. 2008, four years ago. The Post-it note still there on page 86.

211.

I rest my hands on the keys.

It has been a while.

212.

When the sun's fire drops into the Pacific, I uncork a bottle of wine, the aroma intense, like my grandfather's crushed black grapes. His own wine so pungent the color was nearly blue.

The close of another day, one more.

Keep me open to accept the way forward.

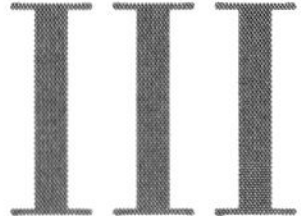

Allegro con brio

lively, cheerfully, with brightness

213.

He has your blue eyes, your intellect.
He makes me laugh, this giant, gentle man.
He, too, is a musician. Though not like you.
Yes, he is a man.
Still, darling, I believe you would approve.

214.

Nine months, to the day, there is Paul. I summoned him. I tell him this and he laughs and says, well, what would be the chance otherwise? Exactly what is it that I conjured, he wants to know, smiling, his body confident, strong, well-lived beside me. At fifty-one, he is my age.

I do not tell him, I cannot, I doubt he would believe me, but here is what I thought: that he would be Italian and we'd be guests at a dinner party. He'd be in the kitchen and ask me if I could join him and help him a moment, and I do and we kiss and it is beautiful, and while the others laugh outside in darkness, here everything is illuminated and still, though I had long asked, *Will there be another?*

215.

He springs from the shower, a towel about his waist, reciting Dante—the first canto of *The Inferno*—from memory, waving his arms. Finished, he becomes the grizzled priest of his high school years in Milan, scolding *Non va bene!* and insisting on another repetition, which *Allora!* he begins comically anew.

Nel mezzo del cammin di nostra vita
mi ritrovai per una selva oscura,
ché la diritta via era smarrita . . .

When I had journeyed half of our life's way
I found myself within a shadowed forest
For I had lost the path that does not stray . . .

216.

Fly, my darling, Lyn wrote me in a final birthday card, two months before the end. And I am curled on the bed, laughing, invigorated by his brilliance, the gentleness of our lovemaking. He calls me *Bella*. He calls me *Cara*. He flops on the bed, and I wrap my bare legs about him.

"I did summon you, you know."

"I know," he says, carefully considering the thought.

217.

It is late, and the arrival of music in this room I once shared with Lyn stuns me. I slide my body against his, transfixed. Cross genre, orchestrally complex, the tones are clear—yet muffled—entering the room as if flowing through a tunnel. *As if coming from the other side.*

"Do you hear it?"

He reaches out, finds my hand, whispers back: "Hear what?"

218.

A morning, only weeks later, his white hair deliciously wild, he bends down, his lips to mine, and whispers that he will (of course) return that evening. And then he doesn't. Days later he calls. His ex-girl showed up at his place and he let her in. He loves us both, he says, and his head is spinning and *he needs some time.*

Time? But there is only this day, only this moment.

Lyn, my love, you taught me that.

219.

I am in the hills of Vermont, at an adult piano camp. I've traveled to this forested landscape for one week, to touch art, to learn again.

I wander through the building's lower level and find a Steinway in a small, wood-paneled room. On the bench: Ravel's *Pavane for a Dead Princess,* a haunting piece I once studied. I remember the opening being relatively manageable, the subsequent passages foreboding. One had to keep the base pulsing—steady and subdued—beneath an increasingly complex tonal melody.

I place the music on the piano and begin. Grief, re-empowered, rises to the surface with volcanic force, its weight flattening each sound. "She's dead," a wildly bearded instructor calls from the doorway. "Ravel's princess. She's not dying. It's done." He joins me on the bench and begins masterfully. I wilt. "It's a different feel. Do you hear it?"

220.

The next afternoon, in the building's rustic, sun-filled salon, the same instructor. "Let layers and textures breathe," he croons to the twenty or so of us gathered around him. "Allow the emancipation of dissonance, the freedom of desire."

The woman to my left is scribbling notes. My pen rests on my closed notebook. I will not forget.

"When we strive to identify a narrative," he continues, "we risk overlooking a rare harmony."

He takes a seat at the nine-foot Steinway. "The aim is not placid resolution." He plays Liszt. When he stops, his eyes scour the room. I sense them landing on me. "You see. There are no rules," he says.

221.

Back home, out for a late walk, I hear her calling. In the flashlight's glow, she sits perched atop a soaring palm, *whoo-whoo . . . whoo*, her expansive wings tucked beneath glowing white. We watch each other, together, alone, in the stillness. Again she calls to me, now softly, *whoo-whoo . . . whoo.*

"Is it you?" I whisper.

Days later, in a local shop on a roughhewn table displaying candles and dish towels are pads of paper, wheat toned and sturdy. The one on top says *Hello Darling* in black in a lower corner. I lift it. The pad below has a small etched owl, and says simply, impossibly, *Owl always love you.*

222.

Tell me, can there be more?
Oh, darling. Always. There is always more.

223.

Patience, patience, patience is what the sea teaches.
Patience and faith. One should lie empty, open, choiceless
as a beach—waiting for a gift from the sea.

Anne Morrow Lindbergh, *Gift from the Sea*

224.

I open the door. He's brought his guitar. It suits him.

"I'm not easy," Paul says, "can you put up with me?"

225.

"Blackbird." He picks out the melody, hums along with his happy tune. He doesn't know that it is your soulful rendition I hear, your earthy seduction wallowing within me, the McCartney/Ray Henderson medley I discovered on a DVD in an unmarked box only weeks after you died. I slipped it in my computer and there you were, *you*, the dinner crowd gathered around, your sung *bye, bye* crushing me. He doesn't know. And just now I will say nothing.

An endearing grimace; he's forgotten how it continues. But I hear the chords, you telling me that my entire life, I was waiting for this moment, to be free.

He looks at me. He wants to be good, he says.
(Yes, darling, I love this man.)

And he begins again.

notes

This story is based on my years together with musician, singer-songwriter, and composer Lynda Roth. In its telling, some names, personal identifying details, and locations were altered. Events and people were left out. An occasional scene and its placement in time were modified in an effort to clarify. The story is my truth, faithful to the stutter of memory.

The referenced choral pieces are Lynda's. The "Blackbird" medley mentioned in the final segment can be found here: www.lyndaroth.com/blackbird.

Portions of the book's passages exist (though in different forms) in the following published works:

What Family Taught Me (Santa Monica Review, fall 2011)
Love Ballad (Squaw Valley Review, 2014)
Heard in Room 303 (Orange Coast Review, April 2015)
Neptune Neptune Omega (Months to Years, February 2018)
Flood (Months to Years, March 2019)
The Graduation (Beach Reads, May 2019)

To the many fellow writers and friends who reviewed the early beginnings of this manuscript and encouraged its progress; to the poets at the Community of Writers who urged me on; and to Marrie Stone, Jacqueline Jaffe, Mirella Zolli, Terry Lucas, and Mary Rakow, whose thoughtful edits and enthusiasm nudged the final words into flight:

I thank you.

To Paul, my cherished companion; to my sisters, who were always there, who somehow understood; and to my daughter and son, who upon reading these words for the first time responded with love in abundance:

You are my everything.

about the author

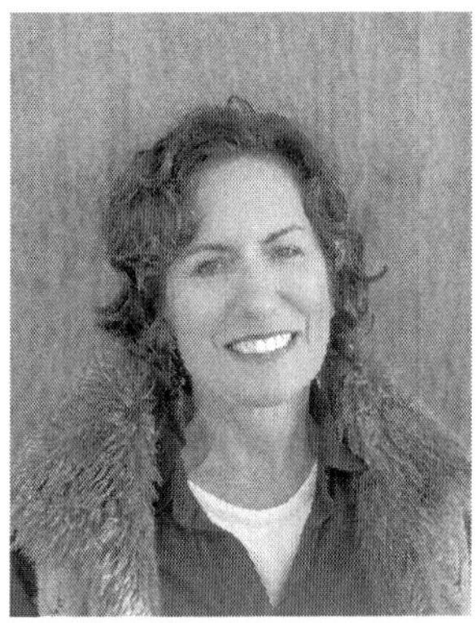

Lisa K. Richter is an American writer and poet. Her prose and poetry have appeared in journals, anthologies, and literary blogs. She holds an MFA in fiction from Antioch University, earned her BA in mathematics from the University of Virginia, and has studied classical piano. Originally from Maryland, she has lived throughout the US and in Europe. She now calls Laguna Beach, California, home.

More on Lisa, this memoir, and her ongoing literary projects at www.lisakrichter.com.

Author photo © Sophia Richter